Mayo Clinic
Analgesic Pathway

Peripheral Nerve Blockade for Major Orthopedic Surgery

Mayo Clinic Analgesic Pathway

Peripheral Nerve Blockade for Major Orthopedic Surgery

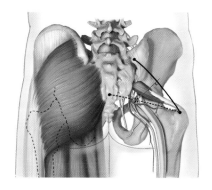

Robert L. Lennon, D.O.

Supplemental Consultant
Department of Anesthesiology
Mayo Clinic
Associate Professor of Anesthesiology
Mayo Clinic College of Medicine
Rochester, Minnesota

Terese T. Horlocker, M.D.

Consultant
Department of Anesthesiology
Mayo Clinic
Professor of Anesthesiology and of Orthopedics
Mayo Clinic College of Medicine
Rochester, Minnesota

MAYO CLINIC SCIENTIFIC PRESS

TAYLOR & FRANCIS GROUP

ISBN 0849395720

The triple-shield Mayo logo and the words MAYO, MAYO CLINIC, and MAYO CLINIC SCIENTIFIC PRESS are marks of Mayo Foundation for Medical Education and Research.

For order inquiries, contact Taylor & Francis Group, 6000 Broken Sound Parkway NW, Suite #300, Boca Raton, FL 33487.

www.taylorandfrancis.com

Library of Congress Cataloging-in-Publication Data

Lennon, Robert L.
   Mayo clinic analgesic pathway : peripheral nerve blockade for major orthopedic surgery / Robert L. Lennon, Terese T. Horlocker.
   p. ; cm.
   Includes bibliographical references and index.
   ISBN 0-8493-9572-0 (alk. paper)
   1. Anesthesia in orthopedics. 2. Nerve block. 3. Postoperative pain--Treatment. I. Title: Analgesic pathway. II. Horlocker, Terese T. III. Mayo Clinic. IV. Title.
   [DNLM: 1. Nerve Block--methods. 2. Lower Extremity--surgery. 3. Orthopedic Procedures. 4. Pain, Postoperative--therapy. WO 375 L567m 2006]

RD751.L56 2006
617.9'6747--dc22   2005053401

Care has been taken to confirm the accuracy of the information presented and to describe generally accepted practices. However, the authors and publisher are not responsible for errors or omissions or for any consequences from application of the information in this book and make no warranty, express or implied, with respect to the contents of the publication. This book should not be relied on apart from the advice of a qualified health care provider.

The authors and publisher have exerted efforts to ensure that drug selection and dosage set forth in this text are in accordance with current recommendations and practice at the time of publication. However, in view of ongoing research, changes in government regulations, and the constant flow of information relating to drug therapy and drug reactions, the reader is urged to check the package insert for each drug for any change in indications and dosage and for added warnings and precautions. This is particularly important when the recommended agent is a new or infrequently employed drug.

Some drugs and medical devices presented in this publication have Food and Drug Administration (FDA) clearance for limited use in restricted research settings. It is the responsibility of the health care providers to ascertain the FDA status of each drug or device planned for use in their clinical practice.

TABLE OF CONTENTS

FOREWORD

Despite the explosion of new techniques and technologies, the single most important change in my practice in the past several years has been the introduction of perioperative regional block protocols. The entire perioperative experience for patients having hip and knee arthroplasty has been improved because of this multidisciplinary approach. Undoubtedly, this approach will be shown to lead to significantly lower narcotic use, a more benign postoperative course with fewer medical complications, lower overall hospital costs, and higher patient satisfaction. These results will lead to the expectation, by patients and physicians, that these block protocols are included in the standard of care. I am indebted to my anesthesia colleagues for the hard work that is required each and every day to make these protocols work for patients. As a surgeon, I undoubtedly receive far more of the credit and gratitude from my patients than deserved.

Arlen D. Hanssen, M.D.
Consultant, Department of Orthopedic Surgery, Mayo Clinic
Professor of Orthopedics, Mayo Clinic College of Medicine
Rochester, Minnesota

PREFACE

"Regional anesthesia has come to stay." These words by surgeon William J. Mayo, M.D., opened the foreword to *Regional Anesthesia: Its Technic and Clinical Application*, by Gaston Labat, M.D. Published in 1922, Labat's text popularized regional anesthesia in the United States by describing techniques already familiar to European surgeons and anesthesiologists. Importantly, Labat described the use of infiltration and peripheral, plexus, and splanchnic blockade (using cocaine and procaine) for head and neck, intrathoracic, intra-abdominal, and extremity surgery. The techniques of peripheral neural blockade were developed early in the history of anesthesia, and over time neuraxial and general anesthesia, with their improved safety, supplanted their use.

Recently, the introduction of long-acting local anesthetics and adjuvants, the refinement of imaging methods to facilitate neural localization, and innovations in equipment technology, including stimulating needles, catheters, and portable infusion devices, have increased the success rate and popularity of peripheral blockade. Undoubtedly, peripheral nerve blocks represent a new era in regional anesthesia and analgesia. Competence in these techniques is crucial to future practice models. However, adequate training and proficiency affect utilization. A nationwide survey reported that 98% of anesthesiologists perform peripheral techniques but most perform fewer than five per month (although the majority predict increased use in the future). Likewise, despite improvements in needle and catheter technology and neural localization, these blocks often remain underutilized and challenging. Studies evaluating proficiency in technical skills have noted that regional anesthetic procedures are significantly more difficult to learn than the basic manual skills necessary for general anesthetic procedures, such as intubation and arterial cannulation. Also, the majority of resident training programs do not provide formal instruction in peripheral blockade.

In 2003, a multidisciplinary group of surgeons, anesthesiologists, nurses, pharmacists, and physical therapists implemented the Mayo Clinic total joint analgesic pathway, a multimodal approach that utilized peripheral regional techniques and *oral* analgesics (no long-acting or intravenous opioids were administered). The results were truly remarkable. With the use of strict dismissal criteria, 95% of patients undergoing total knee arthroplasty and 80% of patients undergoing total hip arthroplasty could be dismissed in less than 48 hours. Importantly, 90% of patients were dismissed to home rather than to a rehabilitation facility. These results were the impetus for the creation of our text.

This book is a practical guide in the application, performance, and management of lower extremity peripheral regional techniques. Labat noted that "The practice of regional anesthesia is an art. It requires special knowledge of anatomy, skill in the performance of its various procedures, experience in the method of handling patients, and gentleness in the execution of surgical procedures." In concordance, we have included original illustrations depicting the surface and internal anatomy for lower extremity blockade, including figures that show the positions of the patient and the proceduralist. The techniques are described in detail, including needle redirection cues based on the associated bony, vascular, and neural structures. In addition, because the perioperative management of patients undergoing major lower extremity surgery necessitates a team approach, instructions for care of peripheral catheters, the dosing regimens of oral analgesics, and the implications of antithrombotic medications are provided. This book is not intended to be a comprehensive text of peripheral nerve block. Rather, the clinician is encouraged to consult the recommended reading lists at the ends of chapters (which include both classic and alternative regional techniques) and anatomical texts, sections, and simulators.

We extend our appreciation and gratitude to the members of the Section of Orthopedic Anesthesia and the Department of Orthopedic Surgery for their collegiality in developing this project, to Duane K. Rorie, M.D., Ph.D., for his meticulous anatomical dissections and instruction, to Mr. Stephen N. Boyd and Ms. Joan Beck for the skillful execution of the original illustrations, and to the nursing staff for providing the highest level of care in the operating suite, hospital ward, and the hospital pain service.

Finally, although over the years the art and science of regional anesthesia have been supported and advanced by countless men and women, we dedicate this book to the two visionaries who brought these techniques to Mayo Clinic: William J. Mayo, M.D., who stated, "Regional anesthesia has come to stay," and Gaston Labat, M.D., who made it so.

Robert L. Lennon, D.O.
Terese T. Horlocker, M.D.

Recommended Reading

Hadzic A, Vloka JD, Kuroda MM, Koorn R, Birnbach DJ. The practice of peripheral nerve blocks in the United States: a national survey. Reg Anesth Pain Med. 1998;23:241-6.

Konrad C, Schupfer G, Wietlisbach M, Gerber H. Learning manual skills in anesthesiology: Is there a recommended number of cases for anesthetic procedures? Anesth Analg. 1998;86:635-9.

Labat G. Regional anesthesia: its technic and clinical application. Philadelphia: WB Saunders Company; 1922.

Pagnano MW, Trousdale RT, Hanssen AD, Lewallen DG, Hebl JR, Kopp SL, et al. A comprehensive regional anesthesia protocol markedly improves patient care and facilitates early discharge after total knee and total hip arthroplasty. Abstract No. SE043. Read at the 2005 annual meeting of the American Academy of Orthopaedic Surgeons, Washington, DC, February 23 to 27, 2005. Abstract available from http://www.aaos.org.

REGIONAL ANESTHESIA AND MAYO CLINIC
A BRIEF HISTORY

Both William J. Mayo, M.D., and Charles H. Mayo, M.D., used local infiltration anesthesia from the inception of Saint Marys Hospital in September 1889. By January 1901, local anesthesia was used in about 7% of the surgical cases at the hospital. In 1920, Dr. Charles H. Mayo visited with a surgical colleague, Victor Pauchet, M.D., in France. Pauchet was a master of regional anesthetic blocks and had taught these techniques to his student Gaston Labat, M.D. Mayo recruited Labat to come to Rochester, Minnesota, and teach regional anesthesia to the surgeons and to write a book describing regional anesthesia.

Labat began his work at Mayo Clinic on October 1, 1920. His book, which was richly illustrated by Mayo Clinic artists, was largely a translation of Victor Pauchet's *L'Anesthesie Regionale* and included a new section on the regional anesthetist as a specialist. Before he left Mayo Clinic in 1921, Labat taught William Meeker, M.D., his techniques of regional anesthesia. Meeker likewise taught John Lundy, M.D., those same techniques, and in 1924 Lundy was appointed Chair, Section on Regional Anesthesia. By 1931, approximately 30% of all anesthetics given at Mayo Clinic involved a regional technique.

The Labat tradition of regional anesthesia spread across the United States. Labat's book *Regional Anesthesia: Its Technic and Clinical Application* was a medical bestseller, having several printings and two editions before World War II. Lundy taught Labat's approaches to Ralph Waters, M.D., the founder of the first academic department of anesthesiology, at the University of Wisconsin, Madison. Waters subsequently taught Emery Rovenstine, M.D., who also was mentored in regional anesthesia by Hippolyte Wirtheim, M.D., Labat's partner at Bellevue Hospital in New York City. The American Society of Regional Anesthesia (1924-1942) was founded around Labat and was critical to the formation of the American Board of Anesthesiology (ABA) in 1938. Many questions on the first written examination of the ABA were directly related to the performance of percutaneous regional anesthesia. Thus, the tradition begun in Rochester, Minnesota, spread first to the East Coast and eventually across the nation. Today, this tradition of percutaneous regional anesthesia is alive, well, and innovatively applied in the operating rooms at Mayo Clinic.

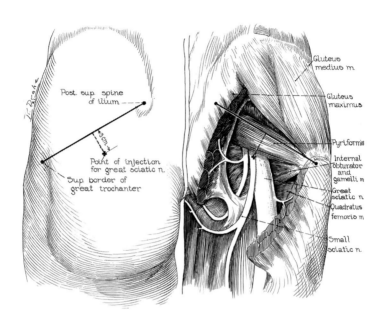

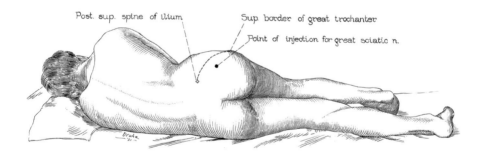

Representative illustrations from Regional Anesthesia: Its Technic and Clinical Application,
by Gaston Labat, M.D., published in 1922.
By permission of Mayo Foundation for Medical Education and Research.

Recommended Reading

Bacon DR. Gaston Labat, John Lundy, Emery Rovenstine, and the Mayo Clinic: the spread of regional anesthesia in America between the World Wars. J Clin Anesth. 2002;14:315-20.

Brown DL, Winnie AP. Biography of Louis Gaston Labat, M.D. Reg Anesth. 1992;17:249-62.

Cote AV, Vachon CA, Horlocker TT, Bacon DR. From Victor Pauchet to Gaston Labat: the transformation of regional anesthesia from a surgeon's practice to the physician anesthesiologist. Anesth Analg. 2003;96:1193-200.

Kopp SL, Horlocker TT, Bacon DR. The contribution of John Lundy in the development of peripheral and neuraxial nerve blocks at the Mayo Clinic: 1925-1940. Reg Anesth Pain Med. 2002;27:322-6.

Douglas R. Bacon, M.D., M.A.
Consultant, Division of Methodist North Anesthesia, Mayo Clinic
Professor of Anesthesiology and of History of Medicine
Mayo Clinic College of Medicine
Rochester, Minnesota

MEMBERS OF THE SECTION
OF ORTHOPEDIC ANESTHESIA

James R. Hebl, M.D., Section Head

David E. Byer, M.D.
John A. Dilger, M.D.
Edward D. Frie, M.D.
Terese T. Horlocker, M.D.*
Sandra J. Kopp, M.D.
Robert L. Lennon, D.O.*
Steven R. Rettke, M.D.*
Duane K. Rorie, M.D., Ph.D.*†
Kenneth P. Scott, M.D.
Rungson Sittipong, M.D.†
Laurence C. Torsher, M.D.
Jack L. Wilson, M.D.

---

*Previous Section Head

†Emeritus Member

Principles of Lower Extremity Peripheral Nerve Block

Chapter 1

Neural Anatomy

The nerve supply to the lower extremity is derived from the lumbar and sacral plexuses. The lumbosacral plexus arises from at least eight spinal nerve roots, each of which contains anterior and posterior divisions that innervate the original ventral and dorsal portions of the limb. With the exception of a small cutaneous portion of the buttock (which is supplied by upper lumbar and lower sacral segmental nerves), the innervation of the lower extremity is entirely through the branches of the lumbosacral plexus.

Sensory and motor innervation of the anterior and medial aspects of the thigh are from the lumbar plexus. The sacral plexus provides sensory and motor innervation of the buttock, the posterior aspect of the thigh, and the leg and foot, except for the medial area innervated by the saphenous branch of the femoral nerve.

Lumbar Plexus Anatomy (L1 Through L5)

The lumbar plexus is formed most commonly from the anterior rami of the first four lumbar nerves, frequently including a branch from T12 and occasionally a branch from L5. The plexus lies on the posterior body wall between the psoas major and quadratus lumborum muscles, in the so-called psoas compartment. The L2 through L4 components of the plexus primarily innervate the anterior and medial aspects of the thigh. The anterior divisions of L2 through L4 form the obturator nerve, the posterior divisions of the same components form the femoral nerve, and the posterior divisions of L2 and L3 form the lateral femoral cutaneous nerve.

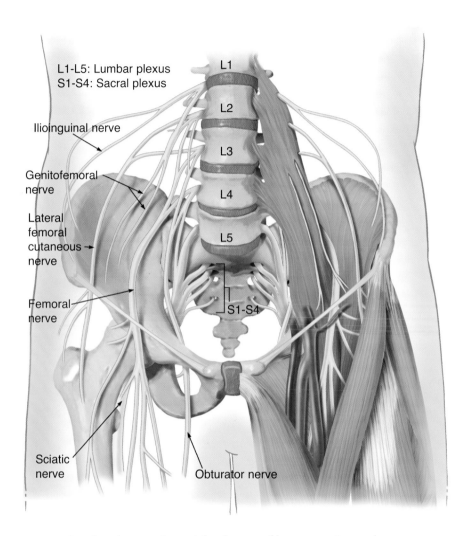

L1-L5: Lumbar plexus
S1-S4: Sacral plexus

L1
L2
L3
L4
L5

Ilioinguinal nerve

Genitofemoral nerve

Lateral femoral cutaneous nerve

Femoral nerve

S1-S4

Sciatic nerve

Obturator nerve

Lumbar plexus; major peripheral nerves of lower extremity are shown.

The branches of the lumbar plexus also form the iliohypogastric, ilioinguinal, and genitofemoral nerves. The femoral, lateral femoral cutaneous, and obturator nerves are most important to block for lower extremity surgery.

The Femoral Nerve (L2 Through L4)

The femoral nerve is formed by the dorsal divisions of the anterior rami of the second, third, and fourth lumbar nerves. The femoral nerve passes through the psoas muscle then emerges in a fascial compartment between the psoas and iliacus muscles, where it gives off articular branches to the hip and knee joints. It enters the thigh posterior to the inguinal ligament. The femoral artery, vein, and lymphatics are in a separate fascial compartment medial to the nerve. This relationship to the femoral artery exists under the inguinal ligament, but not after the nerve enters the thigh. As the femoral nerve enters the thigh, it divides into an anterior and a posterior division.

The anterior division of the femoral nerve supplies the skin of the medial and anterior surfaces of the thigh and also provides articular branches to the hip joint. In addition, the muscular branches of the anterior division of the femoral nerve supply the sartorius and pectineus muscles. The posterior division of the femoral nerve sends articular branches to the knee and muscular branches to the quadriceps muscle. The nerve to the rectus femoris muscle continues on to the hip joint. The terminal nerves of the posterior division of the femoral nerve and the saphenous and the vastus medialis nerves continue distally through the adductor canal.

The Saphenous Nerve (L2 Through L4)

The saphenous nerve is a branch of the femoral nerve. It emerges from behind the sartorius muscle, where it becomes sensory and gives off an infrapatellar branch. It descends the medial border of the tibia immediately posterior to the saphenous vein. At the ankle it crosses with the vein anterior to the medial malleolus and continues to the base of the great toe. The saphenous nerve supplies cutaneous innervation to the medial aspect of the knee, leg, and ankle down to the medial aspect of the foot.

The Obturator Nerve (L2 Through L4, or L3 and L4)
The obturator nerve is a branch of the lumbar plexus formed within the substance of the psoas muscle from the anterior division of the second, third, and fourth lumbar nerves. The divergence of the obturator nerve from the femoral nerve begins as they emerge from the substance of the psoas muscle. At the level of the inguinal ligament, the obturator nerve lies deep and medial relative to the femoral nerve and is separated from it by several fascial compartments. It enters the thigh through the obturator canal.

As the nerve passes through the obturator canal, it gives off anterior and posterior branches. The anterior branch supplies an articular branch to the hip and anterior adductor muscles and provides cutaneous innervation to the lower medial aspect of the thigh. The posterior branch supplies the deep adductor muscles and often an articular branch to the knee joint.

The Accessory Obturator Nerve (L3 and L4)
The accessory obturator nerve is present in about a third of cases (8%-29% of bodies) and sends a branch to the hip joint. When the accessory obturator nerve is not present (71%-92% of cases), the posterior branch of the obturator nerve also sends a branch to the hip joint. The accessory obturator originates at the medial border of the psoas, gives off a communicating branch to the anterior division of the obturator nerve, crosses the superior pubis ramus, and supplies branches to the pectineus muscle and to the hip joint.

The Lateral Femoral Cutaneous Nerve (L2 and L3)
The lateral femoral cutaneous nerve is formed by union of fibers from the posterior division of the anterior primary rami of L2 and L3. It emerges from the lateral border of the psoas major below the iliolumbar ligament and passes around the iliac fossa on the surface of the iliacus muscle deep to the iliac fascia. Above the inguinal ligament, it slopes forward and lies inside the fibrous tissue of the iliac fascia. It perforates the inguinal ligament approximately 1 to 2 cm medially and caudad from the anterior superior iliac crest as it enters the thigh. The lateral femoral cutaneous nerve supplies the parietal peritoneum of the iliac fascia and the skin over a widely variable aspect of the lateral and anterior thigh.

Sacral Plexus Anatomy (L4 and L5, S1 Through S3)

The sacral plexus is formed within the pelvis by the merger of the ventral rami of L4 and L5 and S1-3 or S1-4. These nerves pass together through the pelvis and the greater sciatic foramen. The sacral plexus provides motor and sensory innervation to portions of the entire lower extremity including the hip, knee, and ankle. Its most important components are the posterior cutaneous and the sciatic nerves and their terminal branches.

The Posterior Femoral Cutaneous Nerve (S1 Through S3)

The posterior femoral cutaneous nerve is a purely sensory nerve derived from the anterior rami of S1 through S3. It travels with the sciatic nerve out of the pelvis and into the upper aspect of the thigh. It emerges from the lower edge of the gluteus maximus to lie in midline subcutaneous tissue and continues down the posterior aspect of the thigh and the leg, giving off femoral and sural branches (sensory branches to the back of the thigh and the calf). It becomes superficial in the midline near the popliteal fossa, where its terminal branches often anastomose with the sural nerve. The terminal branches of the posterior femoral cutaneous nerve may provide cutaneous innervation as distal as the heel.

The Sciatic Nerve (L4 and L5, S1 Through S3)

The lumbosacral trunk (L4-L5) and anterior divisions of the sacral plexus (S1-S3) merge to form the tibial nerve, and the posterior divisions merge to form the common peroneal nerve. These two large mixed nerves of the sacral plexus are initially bound together by connective tissue to form the sciatic nerve. At this level, the tibial component is medial and anterior, and the common peroneal component is lateral and slightly posterior.

The sciatic nerve exits the pelvis by way of the greater sciatic notch below the piriformis muscle. At this level, the superior gluteal artery is immediately superior and medial to the sciatic nerve. As it enters the thigh and descends toward the popliteal fossa, it is posterior to the lesser trochanter of the femur on the posterior surface of the adductor magnus muscle within the posterior medial thigh compartment deep to the biceps femoris. At the upper aspect of the popliteal fossa, the sciatic nerve lies posterior and lateral to the popliteal vessels. Here the nerve usually divides into its terminal component nerves, the tibial and common peroneal nerves. The tibial and peroneal components provide complete sensory and motor innervation of the entire leg and foot, except for the medial aspect innervated by the saphenous branch of the femoral nerve.

The Tibial Nerve (L4 and L5, S1 Through S3)

In the lower popliteal fossa, the tibial nerve sends branches to the major ankle plantar flexors, the gastrocnemius and soleus muscles. The tibial nerve becomes the posterior tibial nerve at the lower border of the popliteus muscle. It continues distally between the heads of the gastrocnemius muscles on the posterior surface of the tibialis posterior muscle, along with the posterior tibial vessels. In the lower third of the leg it lies immediately below the deep fascia and next to the tibial bone. The tibial nerve ends posterior to the medial malleolus (and posterior to the posterior tibial artery), dividing into terminal branches, the medial and lateral plantar nerves. The digital nerves to the medial three and one-half toes are supplied by the medial plantar nerve, and those of the lateral one and one-half toes are supplied by the lateral plantar nerve.

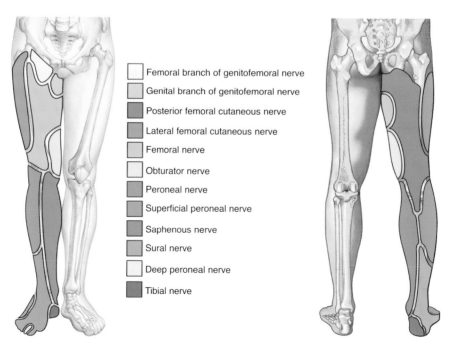

Femoral branch of genitofemoral nerve

Genital branch of genitofemoral nerve

Posterior femoral cutaneous nerve

Lateral femoral cutaneous nerve

Femoral nerve

Obturator nerve

Peroneal nerve

Superficial peroneal nerve

Saphenous nerve

Sural nerve

Deep peroneal nerve

Tibial nerve

Sensory distribution of the lower extremity.

The Common Peroneal Nerve (L4 and L5, S1 and S2)

The common peroneal nerve is the smaller (about half the diameter of the tibial nerve) of the two terminal branches of the sciatic nerve. It descends from the apex of the popliteal fossa toward the lateral head of the gastrocnemius, obliquely crossing the medial border of the biceps. It lies subcutaneously just behind the fibular head. It winds around the neck of the fibula, deep to the peroneus longus, and divides into its terminal branches, the deep peroneal and superficial peroneal nerves.

The deep peroneal nerve continues distally, accompanied by the anterior tibial artery, on the interosseus membrane. The nerve and artery emerge on the dorsum of the foot between the extensor hallucis longus and tibialis anterior tendons. At this level, the deep peroneal nerve is lateral to the dorsalis pedis artery. The deep peroneal nerve innervates the extensor (dorsiflexor) muscles of the foot and the first web space. The superficial peroneal nerve descends along the intermuscular septum in the lateral compartment, between the peroneus longus and brevis laterally and with the extensor digitorum longus throughout its medial side. The superficial peroneal nerve divides into medial and lateral terminal branches. The medial terminal branch crosses the anterior aspect of the ankle and then divides. The more medial division runs to the medial side of the hallux; the more lateral division splits to supply the adjacent sides of the backs of the third and fourth toes. The lateral terminal branch supplies the dorsum of the foot, then gives two dorsal digital branches, one to the adjacent sides of the third and fourth toes and the other to the adjacent sides of the fourth and fifth toes.

The Sural Nerve (L5, S1 and S2)

The sural nerve is composed of branches from the tibial and peroneal nerves. It arises in the popliteal fossa midline between the two heads of the gastrocnemius, descends down the posterior aspect of the leg, and receives a communicating branch of the lateral peroneal nerve. At the ankle, it descends behind the lateral malleolus and runs along the lateral aspect of the foot and fifth toe. It supplies a wide area of the posterolateral aspect of the leg and the lateral aspect of the foot and fifth toe.

Recommended Reading

Anderson JE, Grant JCB, editors. Grant's atlas of anatomy. 8th ed. Baltimore: Williams & Wilkins; 1983.

Basmajian JV, Slonecker CE. Grant's method of anatomy: a clinical problem-solving approach. 11th ed. Baltimore: Williams & Wilkins; 1989.

Enneking FK, Chan V, Greger J, Hadzic A, Lang SA, Horlocker TT. Lower-extremity peripheral nerve blockade: essentials of our current understanding. Reg Anesth Pain Med. 2005;30:4-35.

Gray H, Williams PL, editors. Gray's anatomy. 37th ed. Edinburgh: C Livingstone; 1989.

Rosse C, Gaddum-Rosse P, editors. Hollinshead's textbook of anatomy. 5th ed. Philadelphia: Lippincott-Raven Publishers; 1997.

The visible human project. United States National Library of Medicine. National Institutes of Health [cited 2005 Jul 26]. Available from: www.nlm.nih.gov/research/visible/applications.html

Woodburne RT, Burkel WE. Essentials of human anatomy. 9th ed. New York: Oxford University Press; 1994.

Chapter 2

Dermatomes and Osteotomes

When peripheral techniques are selected for a specific surgical procedure, it is paramount to consider not only the neurotomes but also the osteotomes and dermatomes. For example, the dermatomal supply of the hip joint typically is from L4 to as low as S2, whereas the bony structures of the hip joint do not follow the same segmental pattern and are supplied from L3 to S1. However, when neurotomes are considered, the obturator and femoral nerves, which originate from L2-L4, supply articular branches to the hip joint. Thus, the entire lumbar and sacral plexuses must both be blocked to ensure adequate coverage of the neurotomes of the hip. The same considerations hold for knee and ankle surgery. The importance of understanding the limitations of each of these blocks is essential to successful application.

The clinician also must bear in mind that there is not only extensive overlap between consecutive neurotomes, dermatomes, and osteotomes but also variability among subjects. As a result, the innervation of a specific site or segmental level cannot be determined with certainty. These principles may explain an incomplete or failed anesthesia, even in the presence of a successful block, in a given individual.

Recommended Reading

Anderson JE, editor. Grant's atlas of anatomy. Baltimore: Williams & Wilkins; 1993.
Enneking FK, Chan V, Greger J, Hadzic A, Lang SA, Horlocker TT. Lower-extremity peripheral nerve blockade: essentials of our current understanding. Reg Anesth Pain Med. 2005;30:4-35.
Rosse C, Gaddum-Rosse P, editors. Hollinshead's textbook of anatomy. 5th ed. Philadelphia: Lippincott-Raven Publishers; 1997.

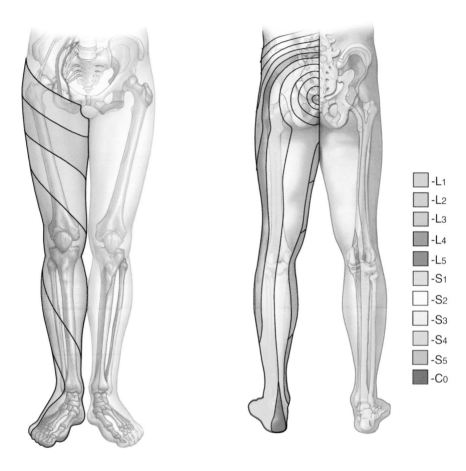

-L1
-L2
-L3
-L4
-L5
-S1
-S2
-S3
-S4
-S5
-C0

Dermatomes and osteotomes of the lumbosacral plexus.

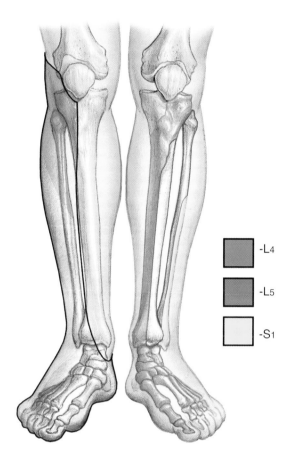

-L4

-L5

-S1

Dermatomes and osteotomes of the leg and foot affected by a sciatic nerve block.

Chapter 3

PREOPERATIVE ASSESSMENT
AND MONITORING

Preoperative Examination

During the preoperative assessment, the patient is evaluated for preexisting medical problems, allergies, previous anesthetic complications, potential airway difficulties, and considerations relating to intraoperative positioning. Overall, patients undergoing major orthopedic procedures on the lower extremity are considered at intermediate risk for cardiac complications perioperatively. However, it is often difficult to assess exercise tolerance or a recent progression of cardiac symptoms because of the limitations in mobility induced by the underlying orthopedic condition. As a result, pharmacologic functional testing, based on clinical history, may be warranted. Perioperative cardiac morbidity may be decreased by the initiation of β-adrenergic blockade.

The patient's medications should be reviewed and the patient specifically instructed on which medications to continue to use until the time of surgery. Specifically, use of antihypertensive medications should *not* be discontinued because of the risk of perioperative cardiac events. Likewise, patients who require chronic opioid medications should be allowed to maintain their dosing regimen. Corticosteroid-dependent patients require corticosteroid replacement perioperatively. Finally, the patient should be queried regarding the use of any medications that affect hemostasis; many patients will have been instructed by their surgeon to begin thromboprophylaxis with aspirin or warfarin preoperatively.

The patient should undergo a focused physical examination. Patients should be assessed for limitation in mouth opening or neck extension, adequacy of thyromental distance (measured from the lower border of the mandible to the thyroid notch), and state of dentition. The heart and lungs should be auscultated. In addition, the site of proposed injection for regional anesthetic should be assessed for evidence of infection and anatomical abnormalities or limitations. A brief neurologic examination, with documentation of any existing deficits, is crucial. The patient also should be evaluated for any potential positioning difficulties (during block performance or intraoperatively) related to arthritic involvement of other joints or body habitus. Hemoglobin and creatinine values are determined for all patients, and other laboratory testing and imaging are done as indicated by preoperative medical conditions.

Ideally, the patient should undergo a preoperative educational session in which the surgical procedure, anesthetic and analgesic options, and the postoperative rehabilitative plan are described.

Additional questions that arise can be answered on the operative day.

Sedation and Monitoring
A sedative is administered during performance of the block and during the surgical procedure to decrease apprehension and anxiety, to provide analgesia for pain associated with the regional anesthetic and positioning, and to decrease awareness of perioperative events. In addition, the administration of benzodiazepines and hypnotics increases the seizure threshold in the presence of increasing blood levels of local anesthetic. It is imperative that patients remain conscious and cooperative during performance of regional blockade in order to provide feedback regarding painful needle or catheter placement or injection. An additional benefit of maintaining patient alertness is the patient's ability to describe subtle motor responses during neural stimulation at a current below that required for visualization by the proceduralist; lower stimulating currents are perceived as more comfortable.

Patients undergoing peripheral blockade should be monitored to allow detection of intravascular injection (heart rate and blood pressure) and adequate oxygenation (pulse oximeter). Because levels of local anesthetic peak at approximately 60 minutes after injection following lower extremity peripheral block, patients should be appropriately monitored for signs and symptoms of toxicity for this duration. Resuscitation equipment and medications also should be readily available. Before the patient is transferred to the operating suite, the degree of sensory and motor block should be assessed. If there is evidence of an incomplete block, the postoperative analgesic medications may require adjustment. Likewise, patients must be immediately assessed on arrival in the recovery room and supplemental analgesics administered early to avoid escalating discomfort.

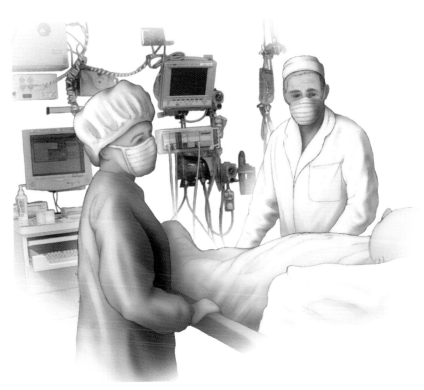

The preoperative block area.

Recommended Reading

Eagle KA, Brundage BH, Chaitman BR, Ewy GA, Fleisher LA, Hertzer NR, et al, Committee on Perioperative Cardiovascular Evaluation for Noncardiac Surgery. Guidelines for perioperative cardiovascular evaluation for noncardiac surgery: report of the American College of Cardiology/American Heart Association Task Force on Practice Guidelines. Circulation. 1996;93:1278-317.

Hadzic A, Vloka JD, Claudio RE, Hadzic N, Thys DM, Santos AC. Electrical nerve localization: effects of cutaneous electrode placement and duration of the stimulus on motor response. Anesthesiology. 2004;100:1526-30.

Chapter 4

Techniques and Equipment for Neural Localization

Historically, lower extremity peripheral blocks were performed with loss of resistance (psoas compartment, fascia iliaca), paresthesia (femoral, sciatic, popliteal), or field infiltration (femoral, lateral femoral cutaneous, ankle) techniques. During the past several decades, electrical nerve stimulation has become the standard method of identifying neural structures. Although there are few studies comparing the efficacy and complications of neural localization with elicitation of a paresthesia with those of a motor response, in general the two techniques seem comparable. Nonetheless, nerve stimulation has become the primary method of neural localization with lower extremity regional techniques.

Nerve Stimulators

The desirable qualities of a nerve stimulator include constant current output (despite varying resistances of the patient's body, cables and connections, and ground lead), a digital display, variable linear output (the current changes in proportion to the movement of the dial), a short pulse width to deliver a precise current or charge to the nerve, and indicators of power or circuit failure. The optimal current with which to begin nerve localization without discomfort and the current associated with "successful" needle placement are unknown. A volunteer study reported that during femoral block, muscle contractions were painful with a stimulating current greater than 1.6 mA. In addition, after elicitation of a paresthesia, the minimal current needed to produce a motor response was less than 0.5 mA in 80% of cases, a suggestion that this may be a reasonable "final" current intensity to seek. However, this may vary between block techniques and in the presence of preexisting neurologic conditions.

Nerve stimulators should be recalibrated periodically to ensure that the dial setting corresponds to the actual current delivered, particularly in the range used for final current intensity (0.3-1.0 mA).

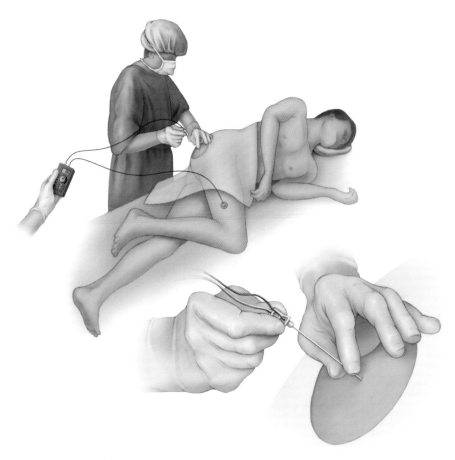

Use of nerve stimulator to localize peripheral nerves and to guide the redirection of unsuccessful needle insertion.

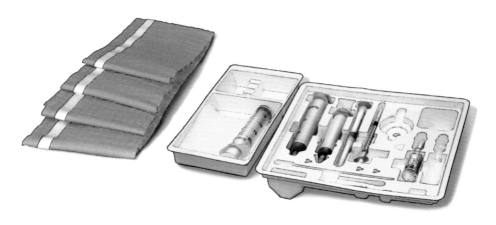

The Mayo Clinic customized nerve block tray.

Stimulating Needles

Both uninsulated and insulated needles may be used to identify nerves with electrical stimulation. However, uninsulated needles disperse the current throughout the entire needle shaft and bevel and require a greater current to elicit a motor response. In addition, the needle *tip* (and site of local anesthetic injection) is likely to not be the area of greatest current density and neural stimulation. Indeed, the needle tip actually may have bypassed the nerve despite ongoing motor stimulation. For these reasons, insulated needles are recommended if electrical stimulation is used to localize nerves. Insulated needles allow a concentrated stimulating current. Needles with a coated or insulated bevel have the highest current concentration and allow for more precise needle placement with less stimulating current to elicit a motor response.

Single Versus Multiple Stimulation Techniques

Multiple stimulation techniques require stimulation of more than one component of a peripheral nerve and a fraction of the local anesthetic injected at each site. For instance, during performance of a sciatic block, a peroneal motor response is elicited first and half of the local anesthetic is injected. The needle then is redirected medially to obtain a tibial nerve motor response and the remaining local anesthetic is injected. Several studies have reported increased success rate, faster onset, and a modest reduction of local anesthetic dose requirements with use of a multiple stimulation technique. However, these advantages must be balanced with concerns regarding the increased potential for nerve injury and patient discomfort. At this time, the efficacy and safety of single versus multiple stimulation techniques remain unclear. However, the advantages of multiple stimulation techniques seem to be more relevant if the purpose of the block is to provide *anesthesia* rather than *analgesia*.

Stimulating Catheters

Traditionally, after identification of the nerve sheath, peripheral catheters were advanced blindly with a stimulating needle or with loss of resistance. However, secondary failure (successful block with initial bolus of local anesthetic followed by inadequate block during the infusion of local anesthetic) occurred in 10% to 40% of cases. The recent introduction of stimulating catheters, which allow continued assessment of the motor response during catheter advancement, may improve these results. Several small observational series have reported a high block success rate and "correct" catheter position with use of a stimulating catheter. Conversely, comparative trials have noted a similar success rate but a higher quality of block and lower local anesthetic requirements with a stimulating catheter compared with a nonstimulating catheter. However, the time needed to place stimulating catheters is markedly longer and there is a potential for catheter breakage because of the repeated manipulations during catheter placement. Also, nearly all investigations report an inability to stimulate all catheters that are attempted to be placed with electrostimulation (yet these blocks are often still successful). Thus, the utility of stimulating catheters, the optimal applications (which regional techniques, approaches), and the cost:benefit ratio require further study.

Imaging Methods

The introduction of high-resolution portable devices has facilitated the use of ultrasonography in the operating suite; numerous studies have evaluated its efficacy for brachial plexus techniques. Lower extremity applications involving the lumbar plexus and femoral and sciatic nerves have been described recently. However, as the depth to the structure being imaged increases, lower scanning frequencies, which are associated with lower resolution, are required. Thus, the existing probes are not well suited for lower extremity (compared with brachial plexus) techniques.

Using ultrasound guidance, the proceduralist is able to visualize the neural structures, needle advancement, and the distribution of local anesthetic during injection. Ultrasonography probably allows a smaller dose of local anesthetic and improves onset time compared with conventional approaches. However, the success rate with ultrasound localization is comparable to that with multiple stimulation techniques, and no data suggest that ultrasonography will reduce the risk of neurologic complications. Also, ultrasonography is unsuccessful for the identification of neural structures in some patients. The presence of obesity or spinal deformities, conditions in which needle guidance would be most helpful, makes ultrasonography difficult. Additional information is needed to establish the role of ultrasound guidance in the performance of regional anesthetic techniques.

Recommended Reading

Choyce A, Chan VW, Middleton WJ, Knight PR, Peng P, McCartney CJ. What is the relationship between paresthesia and nerve stimulation for axillary brachial plexus block? Reg Anesth Pain Med. 2001;26:100-4.

Cuvillon P, Ripart J, Jeannes P, Mahamat A, Boisson C, L'Hermite J, et al. Comparison of the parasacral approach and the posterior approach, with single- and double-injection techniques, to block the sciatic nerve. Anesthesiology. 2003;98:1436-41.

Davies MJ, McGlade DP. One hundred sciatic nerve blocks: a comparison of localisation techniques. Anaesth Intensive Care. 1993;21:76-8.

Fanelli G, Casati A, Garancini P, Torri G, Study Group on Regional Anesthesia. Nerve stimulator and multiple injection technique for upper and lower limb blockade: failure rate, patient acceptance, and neurologic complications. Anesth Analg. 1999;88:847-52.

Hadzic A, Vloka JD, Claudio RE, Hadzic N, Thys DM, Santos AC. Electrical nerve localization: effects of cutaneous electrode placement and duration of the stimulus on motor response. Anesthesiology. 2004;100:1526-30.

Kirchmair L, Entner T, Kapral S, Mitterschiffthaler G. Ultrasound guidance for the psoas compartment block: an imaging study. Anesth Analg. 2002;94:706-10.

Marhofer P, Greher M, Kapral S. Ultrasound guidance in regional anaesthesia. Br J Anaesth. 2005 Jan;94:7-17. Epub 2004 Jul 26.

Marhofer P, Schrogendorfer K, Koinig H, Kapral S, Weinstabl C, Mayer N. Ultrasonographic guidance improves sensory block and onset time of three-in-one blocks. Anesth Analg. 1997;85:854-7.

Salinas FV, Neal JM, Sueda LA, Kopacz DJ, Liu SS. Prospective comparison of continuous femoral nerve block with nonstimulating catheter placement versus stimulating catheter-guided perineural placement in volunteers. Reg Anesth Pain Med. 2004;29:212-20.

Chapter 5

SELECTION OF
LOCAL ANESTHETIC AND ADJUVANTS

Local Anesthetic Solution

The choice of local anesthetic and the addition of adjuvants for lower extremity peripheral nerve block are dependent on the anticipated duration of operation, the need for prolonged analgesia, and the timing of ambulation and weight bearing postoperatively. Prolonged blockade for 24 hours (or longer) may occur with long-acting agents such as bupivacaine, levobupivacaine, or ropivacaine. Although this feature may result in excellent postoperative pain relief for the inpatient, it may be undesirable or a cause for concern in the ambulatory patient because of the potential for falls with a partially insensate or weak lower extremity. A medium-acting agent may be more appropriate in the outpatient setting for orthopedic procedures associated with minimal to moderate postoperative pain. In general, equipotent concentrations of the long-acting amides have a similar onset and quality of block. However, bupivacaine may have a slightly longer duration than levobupivacaine or ropivacaine. Likewise, higher concentrations are more likely to be associated with profound sensory *and* motor block, whereas infusions of 0.1% to 0.2% bupivacaine or ropivacaine often allow complete weight bearing without notable motor deficits. Recent investigations have suggested that increasing the local anesthetic concentration alters the character (i.e., degree of sensory or motor block) but not the duration.

The lowest effective dose and concentration should be used to minimize local anesthetic systemic and neural toxicity. The recommendations for maximal doses of local anesthetics were established by the manufacturers (Table 1). Maximal doses based on patient weight (with the exception of the pediatric population) are not evidence-based. Recommendations for 24-hour doses of local anesthetics also

Table 1. Recommended Maximal Doses of Local Anesthetics

Local anesthetic	Maximal dose, mg
2-Chloroprocaine	800
With epinephrine	1,000
Lidocaine	300
With epinephrine	500
Mepivacaine	400
With epinephrine	550
Bupivacaine	175
With epinephrine	225
	400/24 h
Levobupivacaine	150
With epinephrine	150
	400/24 h
Ropivacaine	225
With epinephrine	225
	800/24 h

Modified from Rosenberg PH, Veering BT, Urmey WF. Maximum recommended doses of local anesthetics: a multifactorial concept. Reg Anesth Pain Med. 2004;29:564-75. Used with permission.

have been established without controlled studies. In essence, the safe dose of a local anesthetic should be individualized according to site of injection, patient age, and the presence of medical conditions that affect local anesthetic pharmacology and toxicity (Table 2). Because of the potential for accumulation of local anesthetic, these considerations are believed to be most critical when large doses of local anesthetics are injected or in association with repeated blocks or continuous infusions.

Table 2. Patient-Related Factors Affecting Local Anesthetic Pharmacology

Factor	Modification of dose
Age	
Newborn (<4 mo)	Reduce 15%
Older than 70 years	Reduce 10%-20%
Renal dysfunction	Reduce 10%-20%, including continuous infusions
Hepatic dysfunction	Reduce 10%-20%, more with continuous infusions
Heart failure	Reduce 10%-20% during continuous infusions
Pregnancy	Reduce concentration due to increased sensitivity to local anesthetics

Adjuvants

Epinephrine

Epinephrine decreases local anesthetic uptake and plasma levels, improves the quality of block, and increases the duration of postoperative analgesia during lower extremity peripheral blockade. Epinephrine also allows for the early detection of intravascular injection. Importantly, concentrations of epinephrine ranging from 1.7 to 5 µg/mL (1:600,000-1:200,000 dilution) reduce the uptake and prolong the blockade of medium-duration local anesthetics to a similar extent. However, concentrations of 1.7 to 2.5 µg/mL have little effect on nerve blood flow, which theoretically may reduce the risk of nerve injury in patients with a preexisting angiopathy or neuropathy. In addition, larger doses of epinephrine injected systemically may cause undesirable side effects in patients with known cardiac disease. Concerns regarding neural or cardiac ischemia must be balanced with the need to detect intravascular injection. In general, because of the high doses of local anesthetics administered during lower extremity peripheral block, the benefits of adding epinephrine outweigh the risks.

Commercially prepared solutions with epinephrine have a lower pH than those in which it is freshly added, resulting in a higher percentage of ionized drug molecules. These ionized molecules do not readily cross the neural membrane, delaying the onset of local anesthetic action after injection. Epinephrine should not be added for ankle block. The addition of epinephrine to local anesthetics with intrinsic vasoconstrictive properties, such as ropivacaine, may not increase block duration but would still facilitate detection of intravascular injection.

Clonidine

Clonidine is an α_2-adrenergic agent with analgesic properties. The effect is most likely peripherally mediated and dose-dependent. Clonidine consistently prolongs the time to first analgesia when added to intermediate-acting agents during *brachial plexus* blockade. Side effects such as hypotension, bradycardia, and sedation do not occur with a dose less than 1.5 µg/kg or a maximal dose of 150 µg. Although the efficacy of clonidine as an adjuvant for lower extremity single injection and continuous techniques is less defined, most studies report a modest (20%) prolongation of the block duration when clonidine is added to long-acting local anesthetic solutions.

Opioids

Although opioids, including morphine, sufentanil, and fentanyl, are often added to lumbar plexus infusions, no convincing data suggest that block onset, quality, or duration is improved when opioids are added to the local anesthetic solution.

Systemic Local Anesthetic Toxicity

Because of the relatively large doses of local anesthetic injected and the proximity of needle or catheter insertion to vascular structures and highly vascularized muscle beds, the potential for systemic local anesthetic toxicity would seem to be very high for lower extremity peripheral nerve blocks. The few cases of systemic toxicity requiring resuscitation occurred shortly after injection, a suggestion that accidental intravascular injection, rather than systemic absorption, is the mechanism. These events also were associated with proximal lumbosacral techniques, such as psoas or sciatic block. Prevention and treatment of local anesthetic toxicity are dependent on the injection of an appropriate volume and concentration of local anesthetic, the use of a vasoconstrictor adjuvant, slow injection with frequent aspiration, and increased vigilance for the early detection of toxic reactions. Local anesthetic levels peak at approximately 60 minutes after injection following lower extremity peripheral block. Thus, patients should be appropriately monitored for signs and symptoms of increasing blood levels for this duration. Resuscitation equipment and medications also should be readily available.

Treatment of local anesthetic toxic reactions is similar to the management of other medical emergencies and focuses on ensuring adequate airway, breathing, and circulation. An airway should be established and 100% oxygen administered. Hypoxia and hypercarbia must be avoided. If convulsions occur, a small amount of a short-acting barbiturate (thiopental, 50-100 mg) or propofol typically terminates the seizure without causing cardiovascular compromise. A muscle relaxant may be needed to secure the airway; although the tonic-clonic motion is inhibited, seizure activity may still persist. Although most toxic reactions are limited to the central nervous system, cardiovascular collapse with refractory ventricular fibrillation may occur, especially with bupivacaine. Sustained cardiopulmonary resuscitation with repeated cardioversion and high doses of epinephrine may be required for circulatory support.

Recommended Reading

Auroy Y, Benhamou D, Bargues L, Ecoffey C, Falissard B, Mercier FJ, et al, the SOS Regional Anesthesia Hotline Service. Major complications of regional anesthesia in France. Anesthesiology. 2002;97:1274-80. Erratum in: Anesthesiology. 2003;98:595.

Enneking FK, Chan V, Greger J, Hadzic A, Lang SA, Horlocker TT. Lower-extremity peripheral nerve blockade: essentials of our current understanding. Reg Anesth Pain Med. 2005;30:4-35.

Neal JM. Effects of epinephrine in local anesthetics on the central and peripheral nervous systems: neurotoxicity and neural blood flow. Reg Anesth Pain Med. 2003;28:124-34.

Neal JM, Hebl JR, Gerancher JC, Hogan QH. Brachial plexus anesthesia: essentials of our current understanding. Reg Anesth Pain Med. 2002;27:402-28. Erratum in: Reg Anesth Pain Med. 2002;27:625.

Rosenberg PH, Veering BT, Urmey WF. Maximum recommended doses of local anesthetics: a multifactorial concept. Reg Anesth Pain Med. 2004;29:564-75.

Chapter 6

NEUROLOGIC COMPLICATIONS

Nerve injury is a recognized complication of peripheral regional techniques. In a series involving more than 100,000 regional anesthetic procedures, the frequency of neurologic complications after peripheral blockade was lower than that associated with neuraxial techniques, and the complications were associated with pain on needle placement or injection of local anesthetic. Risk factors contributing to neurologic deficit after regional anesthesia include neural ischemia, traumatic injury to the nerves during needle or catheter placement, infection, and choice of local anesthetic solution. However, postoperative neurologic injury due to pressure from improper patient positioning, tightly applied casts or surgical dressings, and surgical trauma often are attributed to the regional anesthetic. Patient factors such as body habitus or a preexisting neurologic dysfunction also may contribute.

Although needle gauge, type (short or long bevel), and bevel configuration may influence the degree of nerve injury after peripheral nerve block, the findings are conflicting and there are no confirmatory human studies. Theoretically, localization of neural structures with a nerve stimulator would allow a high success rate without increasing the risk of neurologic complications, but this supposition has not been established. Indeed, serious neurologic injury has been reported after uneventful brachial plexus block with a nerve stimulator technique. Likewise, prolonged exposure or high dose or high concentrations of local anesthetic solutions also may result in permanent neurologic deficits. In laboratory models, the addition of epinephrine increases the neurotoxicity of local anesthetic solutions and also decreases nerve blood flow. However, the clinical relevance of these findings in humans remains unclear. Finally, nerve damage caused by traumatic needle placement, local anesthetic neurotoxicity, and neural ischemia during the performance of a regional anesthetic procedure may worsen neurologic outcome in the presence of an additional patient factor or surgical injury.

Prevention of neurologic complications begins during the preoperative visit with a careful evaluation of the patient's medical history and appropriate discussion of the risks and benefits of the available anesthetic techniques. All preoperative neurologic deficits must be documented to allow early diagnosis of new or worsening neurologic dysfunction postoperatively. Postoperative sensory or motor deficits also must be distinguished from residual (prolonged) local anesthetic effect. Imaging techniques, such as computed tomography and magnetic resonance imaging, are useful for identifying infectious processes and expanding hematomas. Although most neurologic complications resolve completely within several days or weeks, significant neural injuries necessitate neurologic consultation to document the degree of involvement and coordinate further work-up. Neurophysiologic testing, such as nerve conduction studies, evoked potentials, and electromyography, is often useful for establishing a diagnosis and prognosis.

Recommended Reading

Auroy Y, Narchi P, Messiah A, Litt L, Rouvier B, Samii K. Serious complications related to regional anesthesia: results of a prospective survey in France. Anesthesiology. 1997;87:479-86.

Benumof JL. Permanent loss of cervical spinal cord function associated with interscalene block performed under general anesthesia. Anesthesiology. 2000;93:1541-4.

Cheney FW, Domino KB, Caplan RA, Posner KL. Nerve injury associated with anesthesia: a closed claims analysis. Anesthesiology. 1999;90:1062-9.

Fanelli G, Casati A, Garancini P, Torri G, Study Group on Regional Anesthesia. Nerve stimulator and multiple injection technique or upper and lower limb blockade: failure rate, patient acceptance, and neurologic complications. Anesth Analg. 1999;88:847-52.

Neal JM. Effects of epinephrine in local anesthetics on the central and peripheral nervous systems: neurotoxicity and neural blood flow. Reg Anesth Pain Med. 2003;28:124-34.

Rice AS, McMahon SB. Peripheral nerve injury caused by injection needles used in regional anaesthesia: influence of bevel configuration, studied in a rat model. Br J Anaesth. 1992;69:433-8.

Selander D, Edshage S, Wolff T. Paresthesiae or no paresthesiae? Nerve lesions after axillary blocks. Acta Anaesthesiol Scand. 1979;23:27-33.

LUMBAR PLEXUS BLOCK

Chapter 7

Psoas Compartment Approach

Clinical Applications

This technique offers a single injection rather than three separate needle insertions for anesthesia of the entire lumbar plexus. Psoas compartment block is used to provide anesthesia for repair of hip fracture and minor thigh and knee procedures and for postoperative analgesia in patients undergoing major knee and hip surgery. When combined with a sciatic block, the technique provides complete unilateral lower extremity anesthesia.

Patient Position

The patient is placed in the lateral position; the hips are flexed and the operative extremity is uppermost, similar to the position for an intrathecal injection. The shoulders and hips are perpendicular to the horizontal plane.

Landmarks

There are several variations in the needle insertion site. We prefer those of Capdevila in order to optimize localization of the L4 transverse process and to reduce the likelihood of excessive needle depth. A vertical line is drawn to connect the iliac crests (intercristal line). A horizontal line is drawn connecting the spinous processes in the midline. The posterior superior iliac spine is palpated, and a line is drawn parallel to the spinous processes and originating at the posterior superior iliac spine. The distance between the posterior superior iliac spine and midline is divided into thirds. The needle insertion site is 1 cm cephalad to the lateral third and medial two-thirds of the vertical line drawn between the spinous processes and the parallel line to the spinal column passing through the posterior superior iliac spine.

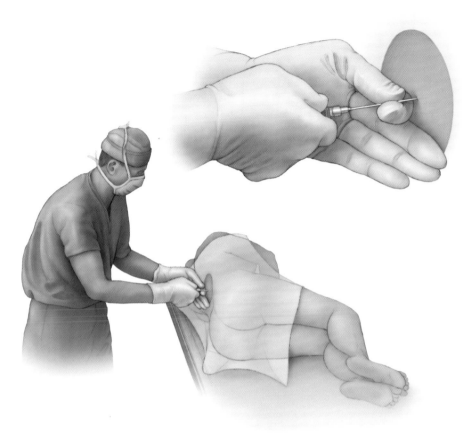

Lumbar plexus block: psoas compartment approach.

Technique

A 21-gauge 10-cm (4-inch) insulated needle is advanced perpendicular to the skin entry site until contact is obtained with the transverse process of L4. The needle is redirected caudad and advanced under the transverse process until quadriceps femoris muscle twitches are elicited. The distance from the L4 transverse process to the lumbar plexus is 2 cm in adults, regardless of sex and habitus. Thirty milliliters of solution is slowly and carefully injected incrementally with frequent aspirations for cerebrospinal fluid or blood. The vigilant proceduralist is acutely aware that negative aspiration does not preclude intravascular injection.

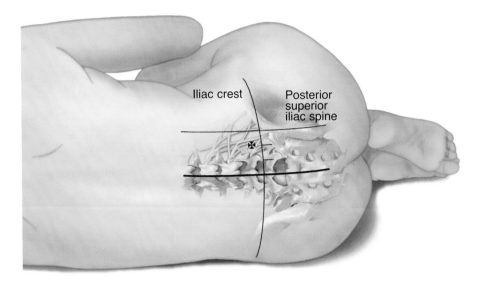

Landmarks for the psoas compartment block. Needle entry is marked 1 cm cephalad to the intercristal line, two-thirds the distance from the midline to the posterior superior iliac spine line. The cross is the site of needle insertion.

Continuous psoas block is performed by advancing a 20-gauge catheter through an 18-gauge insulated needle 5 to 6 cm into the psoas compartment after the appropriate motor response is elicited.

Evoked Motor Responses

The lumbar plexus is identified by elicitation of the quadriceps motor response. Quadriceps contraction is confirmed by rhythmic patellar elevation. Other responses associated with stimulation of the component of the lumbar plexus, such as hip adduction or abduction, also may be used.

Needle Redirection Cues

After contact with the L4 transverse process, the needle is withdrawn to the skin and "walked off" the transverse process by directing the needle slightly medially and caudad to enter the psoas compartment. If bony contact is not made, the needle is directed first caudad, then cephalad. If the anticipated motor response still has not been achieved, the needle is redirected slightly medially, keeping in mind that neuraxial spread is more likely with medial needle placement.

In some instances, motor responses are not elicited but the patient reports light "electrical shocks" down the leg. The nerve roots may have already split into anterior motor fibers and posterior sensory fibers. Only stimulation of the sensory fibers is acceptable and results in successful lumbar plexus block. A needle position that is too deep may directly stimulate the psoas major, producing hip flexion. Of importance, the normal kidney may extend down to L3; thus, if the L4 transverse process is contacted, it is prudent to redirect the needle caudad not cephalad.

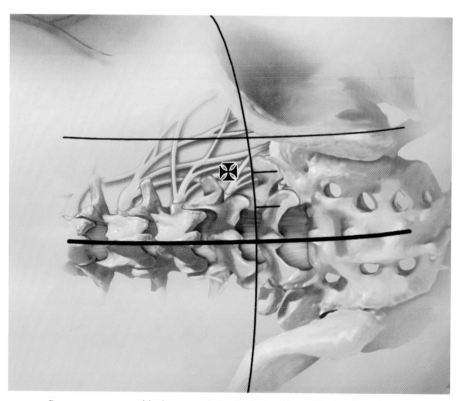

Psoas compartment block: neuroskeletal relationships. The lumbar plexus is identified between the transverse processes of L4 and L5. Dural sleeves extend 3 to 5 cm laterally. The cross is the site of needle insertion.

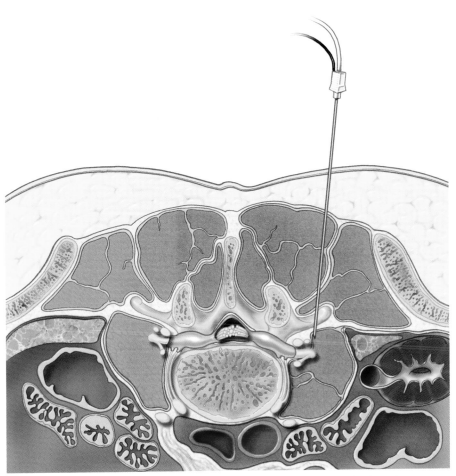

Deep landmarks of psoas compartment observed from above. The lumbar plexus is identified approximately 2 cm deep to the transverse process, between the quadratus lumborum and the psoas muscles. Note the structures deep to the lumbar plexus, including major vascular structures, kidneys, and abdominal contents.

Neural localization with ultrasonography has been described in a cadaver study. The feasibility in human subjects remains undetermined.

Side Effects and Complications

The deep needle placement with the posterior (psoas compartment) approach increases the risk of possible epidural, subarachnoid, or intravascular injection. Epidural or sacral block is reported in approximately 25% of patients. Significant hemorrhagic complications in anticoagulated patients have been reported. The deep and noncompressible nature of the psoas compartment must be considered when selecting an approach to lumbar plexus block; fascia iliaca or femoral techniques may be more appropriate in the therapeutically anticoagulated patient. Peripheral nerve damage is also a potential risk with this technique.

A side effect of the paravertebral approach to the lumbar plexus is the development of a sympathetic block. However, the unilateral sympathectomy is usually of little consequence.

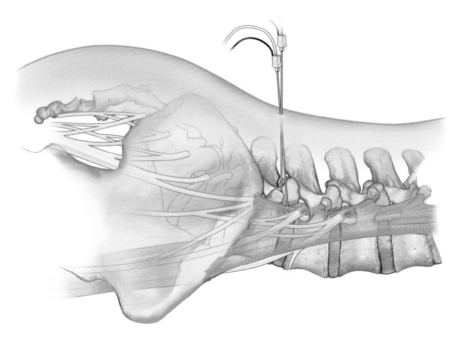

Psoas compartment block: needle redirection. The needle is redirected to pass cephalad to the L4 transverse process or caudad to the L5 transverse process.

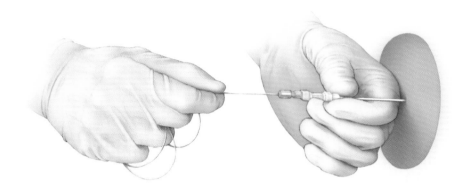

*The left hand is placed against the patient's back to stabilize
the needle while advancing the psoas catheter.*

Recommended Reading

Awad IT, Duggan EM. Posterior lumbar plexus block: anatomy, approaches, and
 techniques. Reg Anesth Pain Med. 2005;30:143-9.

Capdevila X, Coimbra C, Choquet O. Approaches to the lumbar plexus: success,
 risks, and outcome. Reg Anesth Pain Med. 2005;30:150-62.

Capdevila X, Macaire P, Dadure C, Choquet O, Biboulet P, Ryckwaert Y, et al.
 Continuous psoas compartment block for postoperative analgesia after total hip
 arthroplasty: new landmarks, technical guidelines, and clinical evaluation.
 Anesth Analg. 2002;94:1606-13.

Chayen D, Nathan H, Chayen M. The psoas compartment block. Anesthesiology.
 1976;45:95-9.

Kaloul I, Guay J, Cote C, Fallaha M. The posterior lumbar plexus (psoas
 compartment) block and the three-in-one femoral nerve block provide similar
 postoperative analgesia after total knee replacement. Can J Anaesth.
 2004;51:45-51. Erratum in: Can J Anaesth. 2005;52:119.

Kirchmair L, Entner T, Kapral S, Mitterschiffthaler AG. Ultrasound guidance for the
 psoas compartment block: an imaging study. Anesth Analg. 2002;94:706-10.

Parkinson SK, Mueller JB, Little WL, Bailey SL. Extent of blockade with various
 approaches to the lumbar plexus. Anesth Analg. 1989;68:243-8.

Stevens RD, Van Gessel E, Flory N, Fournier R, Gamulin Z. Lumbar plexus block reduces pain and blood loss associated with total hip arthroplasty. Anesthesiology. 2000;93:115-21.

Weller RS, Gerancher JC, Crews JC, Wade KL. Extensive retroperitoneal hematoma without neurologic deficit in two patients who underwent lumbar plexus block and were later anticoagulated. Anesthesiology. 2003;98:581-5.

Chapter 8

Fascia Iliaca Approach

Clinical Applications

Indications for single injection and continuous fascia iliaca block include analgesia for hip arthroplasty, femoral shaft fractures, and total knee arthroplasty. The supine positioning of the patient with this approach is an advantage for patients in whom the psoas compartment posterior approach may be technically difficult (previous lumbar surgical fusion with hardware stabilization or severe scoliosis). The fascia iliaca approach also may be applied when a previously placed psoas catheter has become nonfunctional (positive blood aspiration or misplaced catheter).

Patient Position

The patient is positioned supine, and the anesthesiologist stands on the side to be blocked.

Landmarks

This approach is based on the bony relationship of the anterior superior iliac spine and the pubic tubercle. The anterior superior iliac spine and the pubic tubercle are palpated, and the overlying skin is marked. A line is drawn joining these two points, and it is divided into thirds. A perpendicular line is drawn at the junction between the outer one-third and the inner two-thirds. The needle insertion site is 1 to 2 cm below the intersection of these two lines.

Technique

A 22-gauge 8.75-cm (3.5-inch) pencil-tipped or short-bevel spinal needle is inserted perpendicular to the skin. An initial fascial "pop" is felt as the needle penetrates the fascia lata. A second fascial "pop" is noted after penetration of the fascia iliaca. The fascia iliaca approach is a volume block; on removal of the stylet, 30 to 40 mL of solution (with intermittent aspiration) is injected. For continuous techniques, a 17-gauge Tuohy needle is used. The catheter is advanced 10 to 15 cm beyond the needle tip.

Evoked Motor Responses

No motor response is sought. This is a transfascial compartment block. The essential end point is a two-"pop" (as the needle passes through the fascia lata

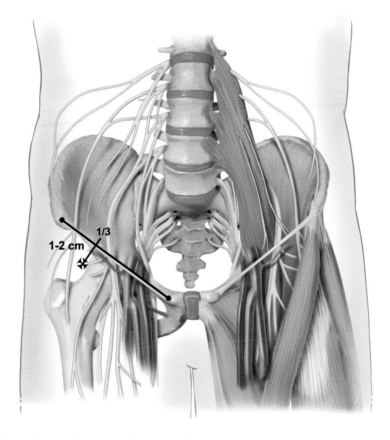

Landmarks for the fascia iliaca block. Needle entry is marked 1 to 2 cm below the junction between the outer one-third and the inner two-thirds of the line connecting the anterior superior iliac spine and the pubic tubercle. The cross is the site of needle insertion.

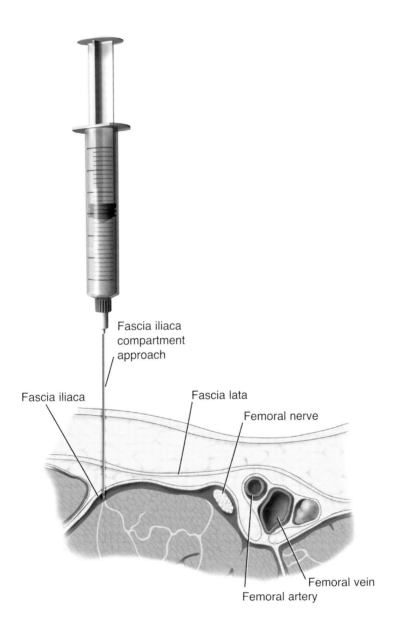

Fascia iliaca block: two discernible fascial "pops" are noted as the needle traverses the fascia lata and then the fascia iliaca. The needle insertion site overlies the hip joint capsule. A third "pop" may signify insertion into the joint space. Note that the femoral nerve is also under the fascia iliaca.

and fascia iliaca) sensation. Alternatively, stimulation with an insulated needle may be used to facilitate needle or catheter placement. Contraction of the quadriceps is sought.

Needle Redirection Cues
Use of a blunt needle (e.g., the Arrow 18-gauge 6.35-cm bullet-tip) exaggerates the fascial "pop" and is useful in mastery of the technique.

Side Effects and Complications
These include hematoma formation, infection, and transient femoral neuropathy; rarely, catheter knotting occurs.

Recommended Reading
Awad IT, Duggan EM. Posterior lumbar plexus block: anatomy, approaches, and techniques. Reg Anesth Pain Med. 2005;30:143-9.

Capdevila X, Coimbra C, Choquet O. Approaches to the lumbar plexus: success, risks, and outcome. Reg Anesth Pain Med. 2005;30:150-62.

Dalens B, Tanguy A, Vanneuville G. Lumbar plexus block in children: a comparison of two procedures in 50 patients. Anesth Analg. 1988;67:750-8.

Dalens B, Vanneuville G, Tanguy A. Comparison of the fascia iliaca compartment block with the 3-in-1 block in children. Anesth Analg. 1989;69:705-13. Erratum in: Anesth Analg. 1990;70:474.

Ganapathy S, Wasserman RA, Watson JT, Bennett J, Armstrong KP, Stockall CA, et al. Modified continuous femoral three-in-one block for postoperative pain after total knee arthroplasty. Anesth Analg. 1999;89:1197-202.

Morau D, Lopez S, Biboulet P, Bernard N, Amar J, Capdevila X. Comparison of continuous 3-in-1 and fascia iliaca compartment blocks for postoperative analgesia: feasibility, catheter migration, distribution of sensory block, and analgesic efficacy. Reg Anesth Pain Med. 2003;28:309-14.

Chapter 9

FEMORAL NERVE BLOCK

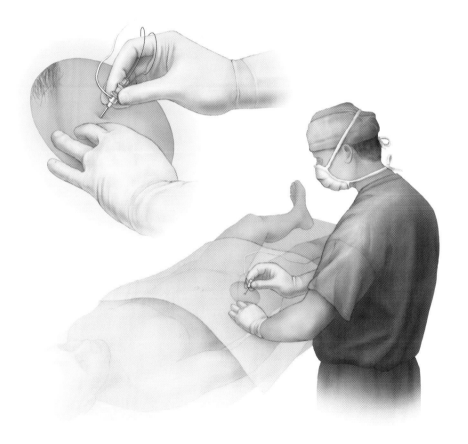

Lumbar plexus block: femoral nerve approach.

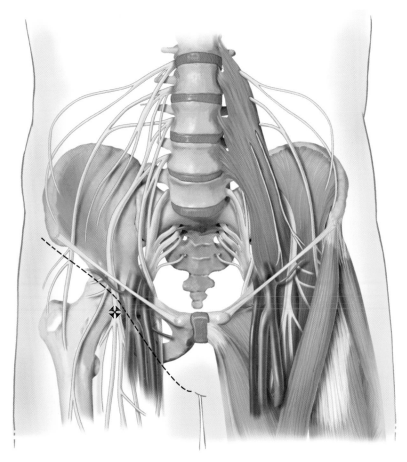

Femoral nerve block: the dotted line corresponds to the inguinal crease. Needle insertion site (indicated by the cross) is 1 to 2 cm lateral to the arterial pulsation at this level.

Clinical Applications

Indications for single injection and continuous femoral nerve block include anesthesia for knee arthroscopy and analgesia for femoral shaft fractures, anterior cruciate ligament reconstruction, and total knee arthroplasty.

Patient Position

The patient is in the supine position. The limb to be blocked is slightly abducted and externally rotated.

Landmarks

A line is drawn between the anterior superior iliac spine and the pubic tubercle, identifying the inguinal ligament. The femoral artery is located and marked just below the inguinal crease. The needle insertion site is 1 to 2 cm lateral to the arterial pulsation at the level of the inguinal crease.

Technique

A 22-gauge 5-cm (2-inch) insulated needle is introduced at a 40° to 60° angle to the skin and advanced. Frequently, two fascial "pops" (passage through the fascia lata and fascia iliaca) are felt. When the needle reaches the depth of the artery, a pulsation of the needle hub is visible. The needle is advanced until quadriceps contraction, accompanied by patellar ascension, occurs. Thirty milliliters of solution is injected intermittently after repeated aspirations for blood.

Continuous femoral block is achieved by advancing a 20-gauge catheter approximately 5 to 10 cm past the tip of an 18-gauge insulated needle. The use of a stimulating catheter may increase the quality of the block and decrease onset time. Additional confirmatory studies are needed.

Evoked Motor Responses

Stimulation of the posterior branch of the femoral nerve is identified by patellar ascension as the quadriceps contracts.

Needle Redirection Cues

Commonly, the anterior branch of the femoral nerve is identified first. Stimulation of this branch evokes contraction of the sartorius muscle on the medial side of the thigh and should not be accepted. Rather, the needle should be redirected slightly laterally and with a deeper direction to encounter the posterior branch of the femoral nerve. The use of an ultrasound probe facilitates locating a nonpalpable femoral artery.

Side Effects and Complications

Intravascular injection and hematoma formation are possible because of the proximity of the femoral artery. However, the nerve and artery are located in separate sheaths approximately 1 cm apart. In most patients with normal anatomy, the femoral artery can be easily palpated, allowing needle positioning lateral to the pulsation. The presence of femoral vascular grafts is a relative contraindication to this block. Nerve damage is rare but has been reported with this technique.

Recommended Reading

Allen HW, Liu SS, Ware PD, Nairn CS, Owens BD. Peripheral nerve blocks improve analgesia after total knee replacement surgery. Anesth Analg. 1998;87:93-7.

Awad IT, Duggan EM. Posterior lumbar plexus block: anatomy, approaches, and techniques. Reg Anesth Pain Med. 2005;30:143-9.

Berry FR. Analgesia in patients with fractured shaft of femur. Anaesthesia. 1977;32:576-7.

Capdevila X, Barthelet Y, Biboulet P, Ryckwaert Y, Rubenovitch J, d'Athis F. Effects of perioperative analgesic technique on the surgical outcome and duration of rehabilitation after major knee surgery. Anesthesiology. 1999;91:8-15.

Capdevila X, Coimbra C, Choquet O. Approaches to the lumbar plexus: success, risks, and outcome. Reg Anesth Pain Med. 2005;30:150-62.

Chelly JE, Greger J, Gebhard R, Coupe K, Clyburn TA, Buckle R, et al. Continuous femoral blocks improve recovery and outcome of patients undergoing total knee arthroplasty. J Arthroplasty. 2001;16:436-45.

Kaloul I, Guay J, Cote C, Fallaha M. The posterior lumbar plexus (psoas compartment) block and the three-in-one femoral nerve block provide similar postoperative analgesia after total knee replacement. Can J Anaesth. 2004;51:45-51. Erratum in: Can J Anaesth. 2005;52:119.

Patel NJ, Flashburg MH, Paskin S, Grossman R. A regional anesthetic technique compared to general anesthesia for outpatient knee arthroscopy. Anesth Analg. 1986;65:185-7.

Pham Dang C, Gautheron E, Guilley J, Fernandez M, Waast D, Volteau C, et al. The value of adding sciatic block to continuous femoral block for analgesia after total knee replacement. Reg Anesth Pain Med. 2005;30:128-33.

Salinas FV, Neal JM, Sueda LA, Kopacz DJ, Liu SS. Prospective comparison of continuous femoral nerve block with nonstimulating catheter placement versus stimulating catheter-guided perineural placement in volunteers. Reg Anesth Pain Med. 2004;29:212-20.

Singelyn FJ, Deyaert M, Joris D, Pendeville E, Gouverneur JM. Effects of intravenous patient-controlled analgesia with morphine, continuous epidural analgesia, and continuous three-in-one block on postoperative pain and knee rehabilitation after unilateral total knee arthroplasty. Anesth Analg. 1998;87:88-92.

Vloka JD, Hadzic A, Drobnik L, Ernest A, Reiss W, Thys DM. Anatomical landmarks for femoral nerve block: a comparison of four needle insertion sites. Anesth Analg. 1999;89:1467-70.

Chapter 10

LATERAL FEMORAL CUTANEOUS NERVE BLOCK

Clinical Applications
Indications for lateral femoral cutaneous nerve block include skin graft harvesting on the lateral aspect of the thigh and use in combination with other peripheral nerve blocks for complete anesthesia of the lower extremity.

Patient Position
The patient is in the supine position and the hands are placed on the chest. The anesthesiologist stands on the side to be blocked, as for a fascia iliaca or femoral nerve block.

Landmarks
The anterior superior iliac spine is palpated and marked. The needle insertion site is marked 2 cm medial and 2 cm caudad to the anterior superior iliac spine and below the inguinal ligament.

Technique
A 22-gauge 4-cm (1.5-inch) needle is advanced perpendicular to the skin entry site until a sudden release indicates passage through the fascia lata. A blunt-tipped needle facilitates appreciation of the "pop" sensation. As the needle is moved in a fanlike pattern laterally and medially, 10 to 15 mL of solution is injected, local anesthetic being deposited above and below the fascia.

Evoked Motor Responses

Because the lateral femoral cutaneous nerve is a pure sensory nerve, a nerve stimulator is usually not helpful for performing the block. Contrarily, Shannon et al suggested that use of a nerve stimulator may improve success if a paresthesia referred over the lateral aspect of the thigh occurs at 0.6 mA at a pulse width of 100 µs.

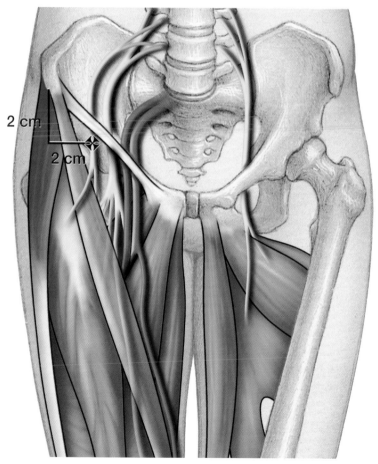

Landmarks for lateral femoral cutaneous nerve block. Needle entry site (indicated by the cross) is 2 cm medial and 2 cm caudad to the anterior superior iliac spine.

Needle Redirection Cues

The nerve also can be blocked by directing the needle in a lateral and cephalad direction to make contact with the iliac bone between the anterior superior iliac spine and the anterior inferior spine. The needle is now medial and inferior to the anterior superior iliac spine, where 10 mL of anesthetic solution is injected in a fanlike pattern. Combining the two techniques increases the success rate; seeking paresthesias usually is not necessary.

Side Effects and Complications

Neuritis caused by needle trauma or drug toxicity is a potential but unlikely complication.

Recommended Reading

Shannon J, Lang SA, Yip RW, Gerard M. Lateral femoral cutaneous nerve block revisited: a nerve stimulator technique. Reg Anesth. 1995;20:100-4.

Chapter 11

Obturator Nerve Block

Clinical Applications

The obturator nerve usually is blocked as a component of regional anesthesia for knee surgery; it is rarely blocked on its own. However, because it is primarily a motor nerve, obturator nerve block can be useful for treating or diagnosing adductor spasm in patients with cerebral palsy and other muscle or neurologic diseases affecting the lower extremities.

Patient Position

The patient is in the supine position with the legs slightly abducted and externally rotated. The anesthesiologist stands on the side to be blocked.

Landmarks

The landmark for the classic approach to obturator nerve block is the pubic tubercle. The interadductor approach also uses the inguinal ligament and the femoral artery.

Technique

A mark is made 1 to 2 cm lateral and 1 to 2 cm caudad to the pubic tubercle and a 21-gauge 10-cm (4-inch) needle is advanced perpendicular to the skin with a slight medial direction. The inferior pubic ramus is encountered at a depth of 2 to 4 cm, and the needle is "walked" laterally parallel to the superior pubic ramus until it passes into the obturator canal. The obturator nerve is located 2 to 3 cm past the initial point of contact with the pubic ramus. After negative aspiration, 10 to 15 mL of local anesthetic is injected. A nerve stimulator is helpful for locating the obturator nerve.

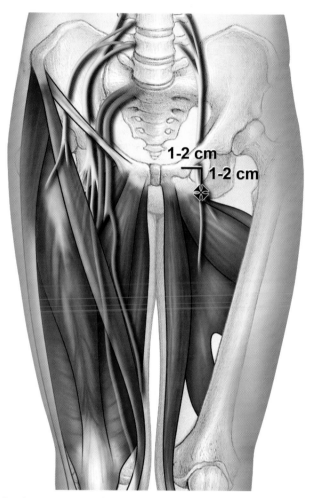

Landmarks for the obturator nerve block. The needle entry site is 1 to 2 cm lateral and 1 to 2 cm caudad to the pubic tubercle. The obturator nerve is blocked in the obturator canal. The cross is the site of needle insertion.

Evoked Motor Responses
The obturator nerve is identified by contraction of the adductor muscles.

Needle Redirection Cues
An alternative interadductor approach has been described. In this technique, the needle is inserted behind the adductor longus tendon, near its pubic insertion, and is directed laterally with a slight posterior and superior inclination toward a mark on the skin 1 to 2 cm medial to the femoral artery and immediately below the inguinal ligament representing the obturator canal. The needle is carefully advanced until contractions of the adductor muscles occur.

Side Effects and Complications
The obturator canal contains vascular and neural structures, and there is a theoretical risk of intravascular injection, hematoma, and nerve damage.

Recommended Reading
Bouaziz H, Vial F, Jochum D, Macalou D, Heck M, Meuret P, et al. An evaluation of the cutaneous distribution after obturator nerve block. Anesth Analg. 2002;94:445-9.

Jochum D, Iohom G, Choquet O, Macalou D, Ouologuem S, Meuret P, et al. Adding a selective obturator nerve block to the parasacral sciatic nerve block: an evaluation. Anesth Analg. 2004;99:1544-9.

Macalou D, Trueck S, Meuret P, Heck M, Vial F, Ouologuem S, et al. Postoperative analgesia after total knee replacement: the effect of an obturator nerve block added to the femoral 3-in-1 nerve block. Anesth Analg. 2004;99:251-4.

Wassef MR. Interadductor approach to obturator nerve blockade for spastic conditions of adductor thigh muscles. Reg Anesth. 1993;18:13-7.

Chapter 12

SAPHENOUS NERVE BLOCKS

Clinical Applications

The saphenous nerve is a cutaneous branch of the femoral nerve, arising in the femoral triangle. It descends laterally to the femoral artery and enters the adductor canal. The nerve exits from the lower part of the canal, emerging between the sartorius and gracilis muscles. The nerve becomes subcutaneous below the sartorius at the medial side of the knee. It descends down the medial border of the tibia immediately behind the long saphenous vein. The nerve crosses with the vein in front of the medial malleolus and extends as far as the base of the great toe. The saphenous nerve supplies an extensive cutaneous area over the medial side of the knee, leg, ankle, and foot.

Saphenous nerve blocks are commonly performed as a component of knee and ankle blocks. Supplemental block of the saphenous nerve is required for surgical procedures to the medial aspect of the leg, ankle, and foot or when a tourniquet or Esmarch's bandage is applied. Patients with thigh tourniquet placement require a more proximal block near the saphenous nerve origin in the femoral triangle. Various nerve block approaches are described, from its origin in the femoral triangle to the medial malleolus.

Saphenous Nerve Block at the Level of the Femoral Triangle

Patient Position

The patient is positioned in the supine position. The leg is extended at the knee, and the long axis of the foot is at a 90° angle to the table. The anesthesiologist stands at the side to be blocked.

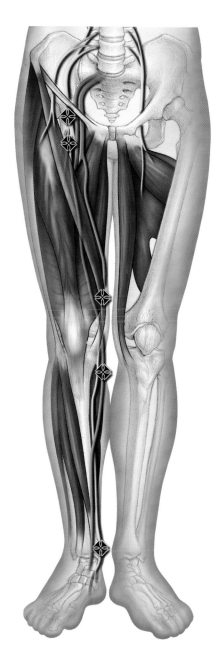

Frontal view of the lower extremity, showing the saphenous nerve.
Sites to block the saphenous nerve are indicated by crosses.

Landmarks

The landmarks are the inguinal ligament, the femoral artery, and the proximal medial border of the sartorius muscle. The femoral artery pulse is palpated and marked. A mark is placed 1 to 2 cm lateral to the artery and medial to the upper border of the sartorius muscle.

Vastus Medialus Technique

A 22-gauge 5-cm (2-inch) insulated needle is introduced perpendicular to the skin at the needle insertion site and advanced until an evoked vastus medialis muscle response is elicited at 0.5 mA or less. A total of 5 to 10 mL of solution is injected incrementally after negative aspiration. Alternatively, a more proximal block of the femoral nerve may be performed if total volume of anesthetic solution is not an issue.

Evoked Motor Responses

The saphenous nerve is identified by elicitation of the vastus medialis motor response.

Saphenous Nerve Block at the Level of the Knee

Patient Position

The patient is in the supine position, the leg is extended at the knee, and the long axis of the foot is at a 90° angle to the table. The anesthesiologist stands at the side to be blocked.

Landmarks

These saphenous nerve blocks are based on the relationship of the nerves to the superior pole of the patella, tibial tuberosity, medial head of gastrocnemius muscle, sartorius muscle, and saphenous vein.

Field Block Technique

A 25-gauge 5-cm (2-inch) needle is inserted above the medial surface of the tibia and 5 to 7 mL of solution is infiltrated subcutaneously in a fanlike pattern. Classically, this saphenous nerve block was performed as a blind subcutaneous infiltration over the medial surface of the tibia (between the tibial tuberosity and the medial head of the gastrocnemius muscle). However, success rates with this technique ranged between 33% and 65%.

Transsartorial Technique
The sartorius muscle is palpated on the medial side, just above the knee. At the level of the upper pole of the patella, a 22-gauge 5-cm (2-inch) needle is advanced 45° from the coronal plane, through the muscle belly of the sartorius, until a fascial "pop" or click is noted (1.5-3 cm). After negative aspiration, 10 mL of local anesthetic is injected. Success rates for the transsartorial approach are 70% to 80%.

Paravenous Technique
Below the knee the saphenous nerve is immediately adjacent to the vein. The saphenous vein is identified by placing a thigh tourniquet and allowing the leg to hang down for at least 60 seconds. Ultrasound guidance also may be helpful. A subcutaneous paravascular injection is performed using a 25-gauge 5-cm (2-inch) needle with 5 mL of local anesthetic on each side of the vein, and care is taken to avoid intravenous injection. The success rate is approximately 100%. However, painless hematomas often occur with this approach.

Evoked Motor Responses
No motor response is sought. Although the saphenous nerve is pure sensory distal to the femoral triangle, the nerve may be localized using a nerve stimulator and eliciting sensory "electrical" pulsations.

Saphenous Nerve Block at the Ankle
The saphenous nerve follows the long saphenous vein to the medial malleolus and supplies the skin of the foot medially, to the midfoot. The saphenous nerve is usually one of the five peripheral nerves blocked at the ankle.

Patient Position
The patient is in the supine position, and a padded table crutch support or pillow is placed under the calf to flex the leg 45° (see illustration on page 93). The anesthesiologist stands at the foot of the patient.

Landmarks
The medial malleolus, saphenous vein, and the needle insertion site for the deep peroneal nerve block are identified. The nerve is located between the saphenous vein and the medial malleolus.

Technique
A 25-gauge 5-cm (2-inch) needle is inserted at the site for the deep peroneal nerve block and directed medially to subcutaneously infiltrate 5 mL of solution around the great saphenous vein.

Evoked Motor Responses
No motor response is sought.

Needle Redirection Cues
A 25-gauge 8.75-cm (3.5-inch) spinal needle may facilitate advancing the needle subcutaneously from the midline insertion site to the medial malleolus. An alternative is to insert the needle above and medial to the medial malleolus and 5 to 7 mL of solution is infiltrated subcutaneously about the saphenous vein in a fanlike pattern.

Side Effects and Complications
There is a theoretical risk of intravascular injection, hematoma, and nerve damage at all approaches to the saphenous nerve.

Recommended Reading
Comfort VK, Lang SA, Yip RW. Saphenous nerve anaesthesia: a nerve stimulator technique. Can J Anaesth. 1996;43:852-7.

De Mey JC, Deruyck LJ, Cammu G, De Baerdemaeker LE, Mortier EP. A paravenous approach for the saphenous nerve block. Reg Anesth Pain Med. 2001;26:504-6.

Mansour NY. Sub-sartorial saphenous nerve block with the aid of nerve stimulator. Reg Anesth. 1993;18:266-8.

van der Wal M, Lang SA, Yip RW. Transsartorial approach for saphenous nerve block. Can J Anaesth. 1993;40:542-6.

SECTION III

SCIATIC NERVE BLOCK

Chapter 13

CLASSIC POSTERIOR APPROACH OF LABAT

Clinical Applications
Because of its wide sensory distribution, the sciatic nerve block can be used, together with a saphenous or femoral nerve block, for any surgical procedure below the knee which does not require a thigh tourniquet. It can be used in combination with other peripheral nerve blocks to provide anesthesia for surgical procedures involving the thigh and knee.

Patient Position
The patient is positioned laterally in a modified Sims' position; the leg to be blocked is rolled forward onto the flexed knee as the heel rests on the knee of the lowermost aspect of the nonoperative leg.

Landmarks
This approach is based on the bony relationship of the posterior superior iliac spine and the greater trochanter of the femur. The dorsal tip of the greater trochanter and the posterior superior iliac spine are identified, and a line is drawn joining these two points. A perpendicular line is drawn bisecting this line and extending 3 to 5 cm caudally, the site of the needle insertion.

A confirmatory line can be drawn connecting the greater trochanter to a point 1 cm below the sacral hiatus. The needle insertion site is the intersection between this line and the line bisecting the greater trochanter and the posterior superior iliac spine line.

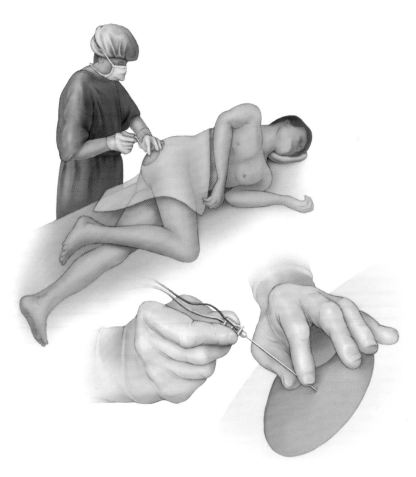

Labat's classic posterior approach.

Technique

Some experts recommend that sciatic nerve block be initiated well before the scheduled time of operation to allow for long latencies.

A 21-gauge 10-cm (4-inch) insulated needle is advanced perpendicular to the skin until an evoked motor response is elicited.

The initial stimulating current should be kept at 0.75 mA or less because direct stimulation of the gluteus maximus muscle with higher currents can mimic sciatic nerve stimulation. Also, high-current stimulation may result in vigorous rhythmic contractions of the gluteus maximus, which are distracting to the proceduralist and uncomfortable for the patient.

Once the needle is properly placed, 20 to 30 mL of solution is slowly, carefully, and incrementally injected. If a paresthesia is elicited on initial injection, the needle is repositioned until an evoked motor response of the foot unaccompanied by pain on injection is achieved with no paresthesia on injection and no blood return on repeated aspirations.

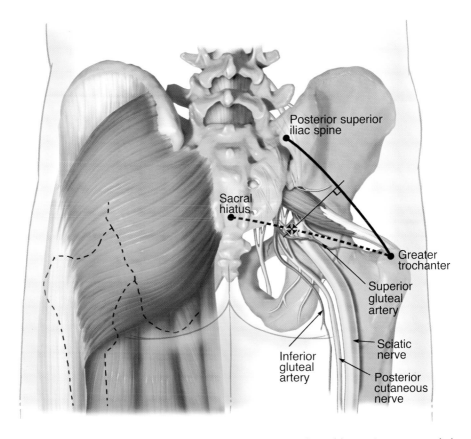

Sciatic nerve block: posterior approach. Needle insertion (indicated by cross) is 5 cm caudad along the perpendicular line that bisects a line connecting the posterior superior iliac spine and the greater trochanter. The superior gluteal artery is immediately medial to the sciatic nerve at this level.

Evoked Motor Responses

Stimulation of the tibial nerve component produces plantar flexion and inversion of the foot. Common peroneal nerve stimulation produces dorsiflexion and eversion of the foot.

Many methods have been tried to improve success with sciatic nerve blockade. Attempts to place the needle in the middle of the sciatic nerve by identifying a specific motor end point (foot inversion) may increase success rates. Another method is the concept of multiple injections. The two major components (dorsiflexion and plantar flexion) of the sciatic nerve are separately identified and blocked.

Needle Redirection Cues

Knowledge of neural anatomy allows the clinician to redirect the needle on the basis of the motor response sought and that obtained. If bone is encountered, the needle is directed medially. If blood is aspirated, the needle is directed laterally.

If knee flexion is elicited as a result of contraction of the tensor fascia lata, the superior gluteal nerve is stimulated. This response indicates the needle is posterior, lateral, and cephalad to the sciatic nerve and should be redirected. Hamstring contraction should not be accepted as a suitable response because it can be due to direct gluteal muscle stimulation.

Side Effects and Complications

The block is technically not difficult to perform. Hematoma formation is possible; nerve damage has been reported, although persistent paresthesias usually are self-limited. A minimal degree of vasodilation may occur with sciatic nerve block.

Recommended Reading

Dalans B, Tanguy A, Vanneuville G. Sciatic nerve blocks in children: comparison of the posterior, anterior, and lateral approaches in 180 pediatric patients. Anesth Analg. 1990;70:131-7.

Labat G. Regional anesthesia: its technic and clinical application. Philadelphia: WB Saunders Company; 1922.

Winnie AP. Regional anesthesia. Surg Clin North Am. 1975;55(4):861-92.

Chapter 14

Parasacral Approach

Clinical Applications

The parasacral approach is the most proximal of the posterior approaches to the sciatic nerve. As a result, the posterior cutaneous nerve usually is blocked, and the gluteal, pudendal, and obturator nerves frequently are blocked. This approach has been used to provide analgesia after major knee, foot, and ankle reconstruction. For procedures above the knee, this approach may provide an advantage over more distal approaches to the sciatic nerve. However, for procedures below the knee, the adductor weakness (from obturator and superior gluteal nerve block) may be disadvantageous for mobilization of the patient.

Patient Position

The patient is positioned laterally with the side to be blocked uppermost.

Landmarks

This approach is based on the bony relationship of the posterior superior iliac spine and the ischial tuberosity.

The most prominent aspects of the posterior superior iliac spine and the ischial tuberosity are identified, and a line is drawn joining these two points. Along the line, a mark is made at 6 cm inferior to the posterior superior iliac spine, defining the needle insertion site.

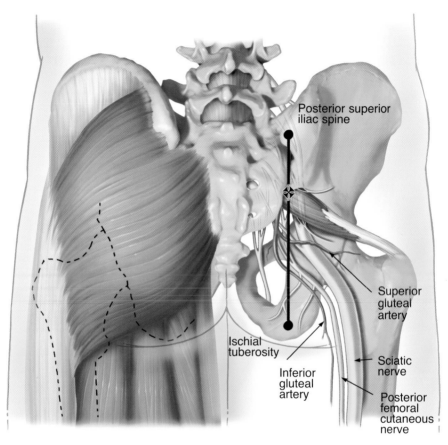

Sciatic nerve block: parasacral approach. This is the most proximal approach to the sciatic nerve and also results in block of the posterior femoral cutaneous nerve. The cross is the site of needle insertion.

Technique

A 21-gauge 10-cm (4-inch) insulated needle is advanced in a sagittal plane until an evoked motor response is elicited, typically at a depth 5 to 7 cm from the skin. Once the needle is properly placed, 20 to 30 mL of solution is slowly and incrementally injected.

Evoked Motor Responses

Plantar flexion of the foot (tibial nerve component) or dorsiflexion (common peroneal nerve) is an acceptable motor response. Because of the proximal nature of the block, a hamstring motor response also is acceptable.

Needle Redirection Cues

If the needle is too cephalad, it may contact bone (ilium above the upper margin of the sciatic notch). The needle should be reinserted caudad 2 to 3 cm along the posterior superior iliac spine–ischial tuberosity marked line. If the needle is directed too medially, the sacrum is encountered.

Side Effects and Complications

This block is not technically difficult to perform. Hematoma formation and nerve damage are possible. Theoretical complications include penetration of pelvic structures with the needle (rectum, internal iliac vessel perforation).

Recommended Reading

Bruelle P, Cuvillon P, Ripart J, Eledjam MD. Sciatic nerve block: parasacral approach [abstract]. Reg Anesth. 1998;23 Suppl:78.

Mansour NY. Reevaluating the sciatic nerve block: another landmark for consideration. Reg Anesth. 1993;18:322-3.

Morris GF, Lang SA. Continuous parasacral sciatic nerve block: two case reports. Reg Anesth. 1997;22:469-72.

Morris GF, Lang SA, Dust WN, Van der Wal M. The parasacral sciatic nerve block. Reg Anesth. 1997;22:223-8.

Chapter 15

SUBGLUTEAL APPROACH

Clinical Applications

The indications for the subgluteal approach are those for sciatic nerve block: anesthesia or analgesia for knee, leg, and foot surgery. Because of the distal needle insertion site, the posterior cutaneous femoral nerve may remain unblocked. This has implications for patients undergoing knee surgery or procedures requiring the use of a thigh tourniquet.

Patient Position

The patient is positioned laterally in a modified Sims' position; the leg to be blocked is rolled forward onto the flexed knee as the heel rests on the knee of the dependent (nonoperative) leg.

Landmarks

This approach is based on the bony relationship of the greater trochanter and the ischial tuberosity. The most prominent aspects of the greater trochanter and the ischial tuberosity are identified by palpation, and a line is drawn joining these two points. A perpendicular line is drawn bisecting this line and extending 4 to 6 cm caudad. The second line approximates the location of the sciatic nerve. The site of the needle insertion may be at the intersection of the two lines or as far as 6 cm distally along the second line.

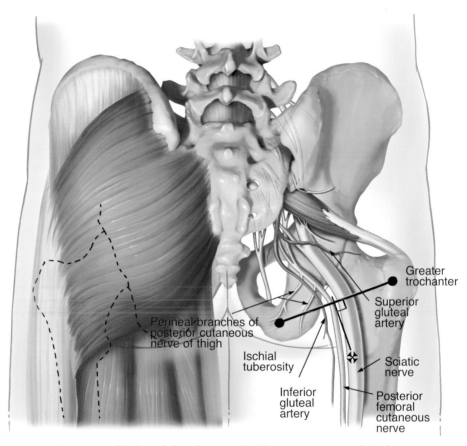

Sciatic nerve block: subgluteal approach. The sciatic nerve is relatively superficial at this level. Needle insertion (indicated by cross) is near the gluteal crease, between the hamstring muscles.

Technique

A 21-gauge 10-cm (4-inch) insulated needle is inserted perpendicularly until an evoked motor response is elicited, typically at 3 to 5 cm. After a tibial or peroneal evoked motor response in the ankle or foot is elicited, a total of 20 to 30 mL of solution is injected incrementally.

Evoked Motor Responses

The target response is an evoked response below the knee; stimulation of the tibial nerve component produces plantar flexion and inversion of the foot, and common peroneal nerve stimulation produces dorsiflexion and eversion.

Needle Redirection Cues

If no motor response is elicited, the needle may be redirected 1 to 2 cm medially or laterally to the original direction of the needle. It may be helpful to palpate or visualize the groove that can be seen or palpated on the posterior aspect of the thigh. If bony contact is made, the needle is withdrawn and redirected medially.

Side Effects and Complications

There is less risk of hematoma formation with this posterior approach. Nerve injury is possible.

Recommended Reading

di Benedetto P, Bertini L, Casati A, Borghi B, Albertin A, Fanelli G. A new posterior approach to the sciatic nerve block: a prospective, randomized comparison with the classic posterior approach. Anesth Analg. 2001;93:1040-4.

di Benedetto P, Casati A, Bertini L. Continuous subgluteus sciatic nerve block after orthopedic foot and ankle surgery: comparison of two infusion techniques. Reg Anesth Pain Med. 2002;27:168-72.

di Benedetto P, Casati A, Bertini L, Fanelli G, Chelly JE. Postoperative analgesia with continuous sciatic nerve block after foot surgery: a prospective, randomized comparison between the popliteal and subgluteal approaches. Anesth Analg. 2002;94:996-1000.

Chapter 16

Anterior Approach

Clinical Applications

The indications for the anterior approach are those for sciatic nerve block: anesthesia or analgesia for knee, leg, and foot surgery. The supine positioning of the patient with this approach is an advantage for patients in whom the posterior approaches would be difficult or painful. In addition, the supine position has the elegance of a single preparation of the patient for combined femoral and sciatic nerve block. Because of the distal needle insertion site, the posterior cutaneous femoral nerve may remain unblocked. This has implications for patients undergoing knee surgery or procedures requiring the use of a thigh tourniquet.

Patient Position

The patient is in the supine position with the operative leg extended in the neutral position, avoiding external rotation of the leg.

Landmarks

The landmarks described by Chelly are based on the bony relationship between the anterior superior iliac spine and the pubic symphysis. The most caudal and most medial aspect of the anterior superior iliac spine and the most rostral surface of the pubic symphysis are identified by palpation, and a line is drawn joining these two points. A perpendicular line is drawn bisecting this line and extending 8 cm distally, the site of the needle insertion.

The original anterior approach described by Beck used the inguinal ligament and the greater trochanter as landmarks.

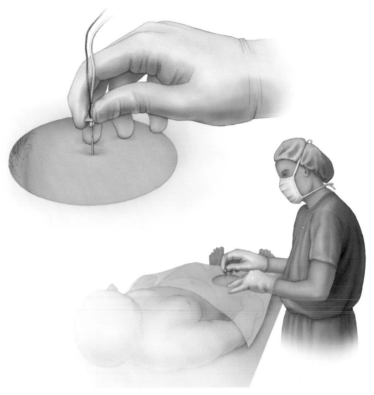

Sciatic nerve block: anterior approach.

Technique

A 21-gauge 15-cm (6-inch) insulated needle is inserted perpendicularly with a slightly lateral angulation. The needle is advanced until it contacts bone, the lesser trochanter of the femur. The needle is redirected medially past the femur until an evoked motor response is elicited, typically 4 to 5 cm deep to the femur. After a tibial or peroneal evoked motor response in the ankle or foot is elicited, a total of 20 to 30 mL of solution is injected incrementally.

The anterior sciatic approach is commonly used in combination with a femoral block for knee surgery. The advancing needle frequently stimulates the femoral nerve at a distance of 3 to 5 cm from the skin. Blockade of the femoral nerve *after* sciatic block theoretically decreases the risk of femoral nerve injury due to needle trauma.

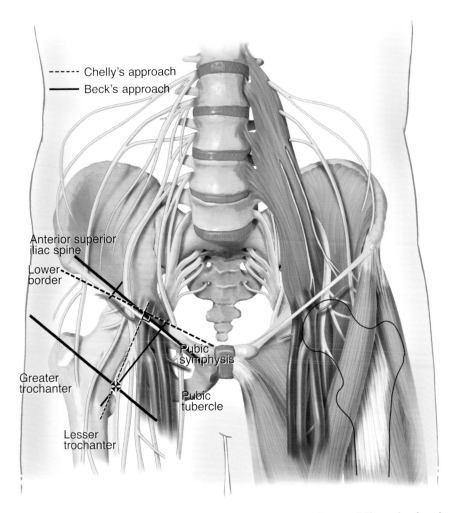

Sciatic nerve block: anterior approach. Two alternative approaches use different landmarks to identify a common insertion site (indicated by cross).

Evoked Motor Responses

As the needle is slowly advanced, the first evoked response is commonly a quadriceps contraction as the needle glides past the femoral nerve. The target response is an evoked response below the knee: stimulation of the tibial nerve component produces plantar flexion and inversion of the foot. Common peroneal nerve stimulation produces foot dorsiflexion and eversion. Contraction of the hamstring muscles is not accepted.

Needle Redirection Cues

Several maneuvers have been reported to improve success with the anterior approach to the sciatic nerve. If bone (femur) is encountered, the needle is withdrawn to the skin, the leg is internally rotated, and the needle is readvanced. If the needle still will not pass by the femur, the process is repeated with the leg externally rotated. If these maneuvers are unsuccessful, the needle is reinserted 1 to 2 cm medially and redirected slightly laterally to advance past the femur. An insertion site 12 cm distal to the anterior superior iliac spine–pubic symphysis line also has been suggested.

Side Effects and Complications

The needle passes near the femoral nerve and artery during advancement to the sciatic nerve. Hematoma formation is possible, and femoral nerve damage has been reported.

Recommended Reading

Beck GP. Anterior approach to sciatic nerve block. Anesthesiology. 1963;24:222-4.

Chelly JE, Delaunay L. A new anterior approach to the sciatic nerve block. Anesthesiology. 1999;91:1655-60.

Ericksen ML, Swenson JD, Pace NL. The anatomic relationship of the sciatic nerve to the lesser trochanter: implications for anterior sciatic nerve block. Anesth Analg. 2002;95:1071-4.

Vloka JD, Hadzic A, April E, Thys DM. Anterior approach to the sciatic nerve block: the effects of leg rotation. Anesth Analg. 2001;92:460-2.

Chapter 17

LATERAL POPLITEAL APPROACH

Clinical Applications

The sciatic nerve block at the popliteal fossa level may be used, together with a saphenous or femoral nerve block, for any surgical procedure below the knee which does not require a thigh tourniquet, such as tibia or fibula fractures, ankle arthrodesis, or hindfoot procedures.

Patient Position

The patient is in the supine position; the operative leg is extended at the knee, and the long axis of the foot is at a 90° angle to the table.

Landmarks

The superior pole of the patella is palpated, and the groove between the lateral border of the biceps femoris and the vastus lateralis is identified and marked. A vertical line is drawn from the superior pole of the patella intersecting with the first line. The needle insertion site is the intersection of these two lines.

Technique

A 21-gauge 10-cm (4-inch) insulated needle is slowly advanced in a horizontal plane between the biceps femoris and the vastus lateralis until the femur is encountered. The needle is then withdrawn to the skin and slowly advanced at a 30° angle posterior to the horizontal plane until an evoked motor response is elicited. After a tibial (preferred) or peroneal evoked motor response in the ankle or foot is elicited, a total of 30 to 40 mL of solution is injected incrementally.

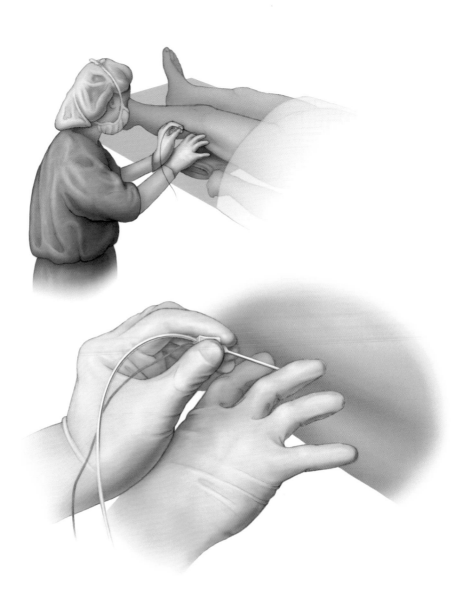

Knee block: lateral approach.

Continuous popliteal block is performed by advancing a 20-gauge catheter through an 18-gauge insulated needle 5 to 6 cm into the popliteal fossa after the appropriate motor response is elicited.

Evoked Motor Responses

As the needle is slowly advanced, the first evoked response is direct stimulation of the vastus lateralis or biceps femoris. At a depth of approximately 3 to 4 cm, the common peroneal nerve (foot dorsiflexion and eversion) is commonly encountered. A deeper and more posterior angulation (45° from horizontal plane) results in tibial stimulation (plantar flexion and inversion).

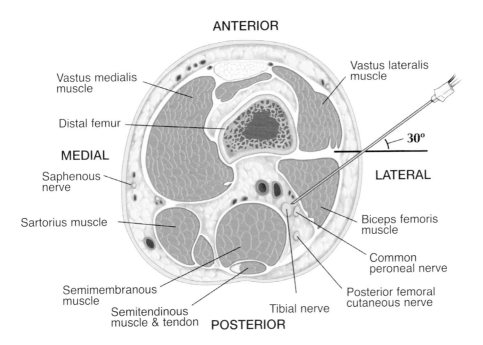

Cross-sectional view of popliteal fossa. Needle position is shown for a lateral approach to the sciatic nerve in the supine patient at the level of the popliteal fossa.

Needle Redirection Cues

Stimulating both tibial and common peroneal nerves has been described, with the local anesthetic dose divided equally between tibial and peroneal components. Aspiration of blood signifies that the needle is too deep and anterior. If neither component is localized, the needle is withdrawn to the skin, the femur is reidentified, and the needle angle is redirected in 5° increments until an appropriate motor response is elicited. Rarely, a more proximal skin insertion site is required.

Side Effects and Complications

Hematoma formation and transient paresthesias are possible. Graft disruption or infection may occur in patients with vascular grafts. Thus, this block is a relative contraindication in patients with indwelling prostheses.

Recommended Reading

Hadzic A, Vloka JD. A comparison of the posterior versus lateral approaches to the block of the sciatic nerve in the popliteal fossa. Anesthesiology. 1998;88:1480-6.

Paqueron X, Bouaziz H, Macalou D, Labaille T, Merle M, Laxenaire MC, et al. The lateral approach to the sciatic nerve at the popliteal fossa: one or two injections? Anesth Analg. 1999;89:1221-5.

Vloka JD, Hadzic A, April E, Thys DM. The division of the sciatic nerve in the popliteal fossa: anatomical implications for popliteal nerve blockade. Anesth Analg. 2001;92:215-7.

Vloka JD, Hadzic A, Kitain E, Lesser JB, Kuroda M, April EW, et al. Anatomic considerations for sciatic nerve block in the popliteal fossa through the lateral approach. Reg Anesth. 1996;21:414-8.

Zetlaoui PJ, Bouaziz H. Lateral approach to the sciatic nerve in the popliteal fossa. Anesth Analg. 1998;87:79-82.

Chapter 18

POSTERIOR POPLITEAL APPROACH

Clinical Applications

The sciatic nerve block at the popliteal fossa level may be used, together with a saphenous or femoral nerve block, for any surgical procedure below the knee which does not require a thigh tourniquet, such as tibia or fibula fractures, ankle arthrodesis, or hindfoot procedures.

Patient Position

The patient is in the prone position; the knee is slightly flexed to facilitate palpation of the popliteal fossa borders and to accentuate the popliteal skin crease.

Landmarks

A triangle is constructed; the base consists of the popliteal crease and the two sides are composed of the semimembranous and semitendinous tendons (medially) and the biceps tendon (laterally). A perpendicular line is drawn bisecting the popliteal crease line and extending 7 to 8 cm cephalad. The needle insertion site is just lateral (0.5-1 cm) to the 7- to 8-cm mark.

Technique

A 21-gauge 5-cm (2-inch) insulated needle is advanced at a 45° angle until an evoked motor response is elicited. The average depth from skin to nerve in adults is 1.5 to 2 cm. After a tibial (preferred) or peroneal evoked motor response is elicited in the ankle or foot, a total of 30 to 40 mL of solution is injected incrementally.

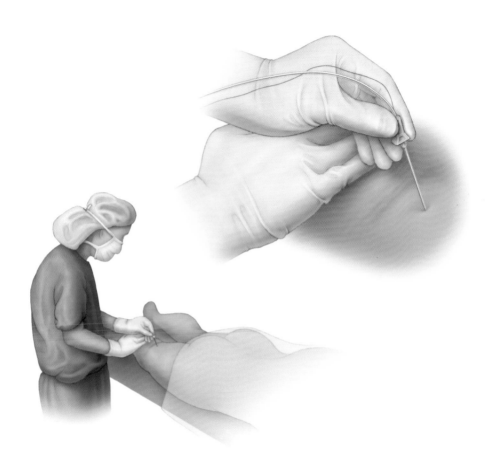

Knee block: posterior approach.

Continuous popliteal block is performed by advancing a 20-gauge catheter through an 18-gauge insulated needle 5 to 6 cm into the popliteal fossa after the appropriate motor response is elicited.

Evoked Motor Responses

Plantar flexion of the foot or toes and foot inversion indicate tibial nerve stimulation, the preferred response. Dorsiflexion of the foot, toe extension, and foot eversion indicate common peroneal nerve stimulation. Attempts to place the needle near the tibial nerve (foot inversion) may increase the success rate.

Alternatively, with use of the multiple injection approach, the two major components (dorsiflexion and eversion, planter flexion and inversion) of the sciatic nerve are separately identified and blocked, and the local anesthetic dose is divided equally.

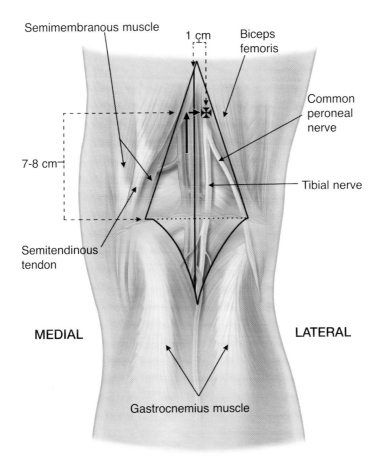

Posterior view of popliteal fossa. Landmarks for posterior approach. A perpendicular line is drawn bisecting the popliteal crease line and extending 7 to 8 cm cephalad. The needle entry site (indicated by cross) is just lateral (0.5-1 cm) to the perpendicular line.

Needle Redirection Cues

If the peroneal nerve is stimulated, medial redirection results in localization of the tibial component. If the tibial nerve is stimulated, lateral redirection results in localization of the peroneal component. Aspiration of blood signifies that the needle is too deep and too medial and should be redirected laterally.

Side Effects and Complications

The block is not technically difficult to perform. Hematoma formation and transient paresthesias are possible. A relative contraindication is presence of a vascular graft.

Recommended Reading

Benzon HT, Kim C, Benzon HP, Silverstein ME, Jericho B, Prillaman K, et al. Correlation between evoked motor response of the sciatic nerve and sensory blockade. Anesthesiology. 1997;87:547-52.

Hadzic A, Vloka JD. A comparison of the posterior versus lateral approaches to the block of the sciatic nerve in the popliteal fossa. Anesthesiology. 1998;88:1480-6.

Rorie DK, Byer DE, Nelson DO, Sittipong R, Johnson KA. Assessment of block of the sciatic nerve in the popliteal fossa. Anesth Analg. 1980;59:371-6.

Vloka JD, Hadzic A, April E, Thys DM. The division of the sciatic nerve in the popliteal fossa: anatomical implications for popliteal nerve blockade. Anesth Analg. 2001;92:215-7.

Chapter 19

ANKLE BLOCK

Clinical Applications
The peripheral nerves blocked at the ankle are terminal branches of both the sciatic (posterior tibial, superficial peroneal, deep peroneal, and sural) and the femoral (saphenous) nerves. The lumbosacral plexus blocked distally at the ankle provides anesthesia for surgery to the foot, including bunionectomy, amputation of the midfoot and toes, and debridement procedures.

Patient Position
The patient is in the supine position, and a padded table crutch support or blankets are placed under the calf. The deep peroneal, superficial peroneal, and saphenous nerves all may be blocked from the same needle insertion site, and an additional insertion is required for posterior tibial and sural nerve blockade.

Posterior Tibial Nerve

Landmarks
The posterior tibial artery, posterior to the medial malleolus, is palpated and marked at the cephalad tip of the medial malleolus. The medial border of the Achilles tendon is identified. The block also may be performed with the patient in the prone position.

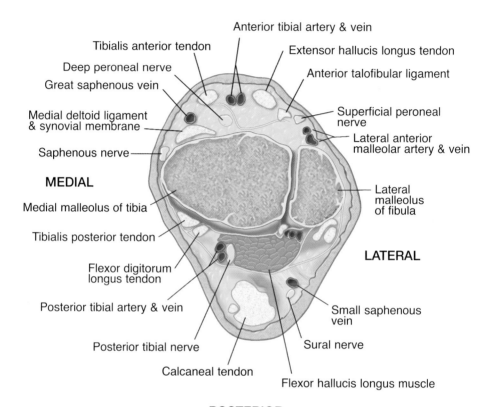

ANTERIOR

Anterior tibial artery & vein

Tibialis anterior tendon

Deep peroneal nerve

Great saphenous vein

Extensor hallucis longus tendon

Anterior talofibular ligament

Medial deltoid ligament & synovial membrane

Saphenous nerve

Superficial peroneal nerve

Lateral anterior malleolar artery & vein

MEDIAL

Medial malleolus of tibia

Lateral malleolus of fibula

Tibialis posterior tendon

Flexor digitorum longus tendon

LATERAL

Posterior tibial artery & vein

Small saphenous vein

Posterior tibial nerve

Sural nerve

Calcaneal tendon

Flexor hallucis longus muscle

POSTERIOR

Cross-sectional view of ankle. The figure at the level of the malleolus shows the distribution of the terminal branches of the sciatic nerve that comprise the ankle block.

Technique

A 25-gauge 3.8-cm (1.5-inch) needle is inserted perpendicularly to the skin at a point 2 to 5 cm cephalad to the proximal tip of the medial malleolus and midway between the posterior border of the upper malleolus and the medial border of the Achilles tendon. The nerve lies 1 to 2 cm deep to the skin. If a paresthesia is obtained, 5 mL of local anesthetic (epinephrine-free) solution is injected. Alternatively, 7 to 10 mL of solution is injected as the needle is slowly withdrawn from the posterior aspect of the tibia. At the supramalleolar level, blockade is

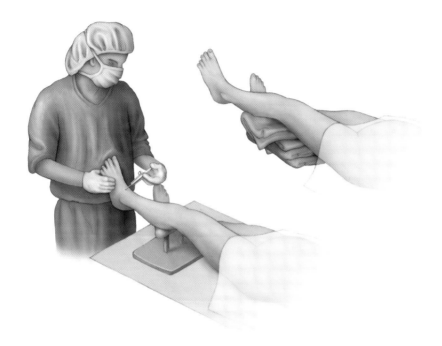

Lumbosacral plexus block at the ankle.

theoretically more reliable because the calcaneal and plantar branches have not divided from the posterior tibial nerve.

Needle Redirection Cues

Stimulation with a 22-gauge 5-cm (2-inch) needle connected to a nerve stimulator may be used to facilitate proper needle placement. The targeted evoked response is plantar flexion. Nerve stimulation may not be effective in patients with a peripheral neuropathy. Ultrasound guidance may facilitate performance of this block.

Deep Peroneal Nerve Block

Landmarks

At the intramalleolus level, the tibialis anterior and the extensor hallucis tendons are identified and marked.

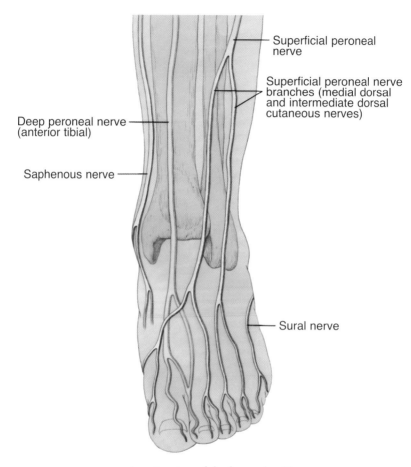

Anterior view of the foot and ankle.

Technique

A 25-gauge 3-cm (1.25- to 1.5-inch) needle is inserted perpendicular to the skin between the tendons. The needle is advanced carefully deep to the fascial plane, and 3 to 5 mL of epinephrine-free solution is injected.

Needle Redirection Cues

If the anterior tibial artery is palpable at the proximal level of the malleoli, the needle is inserted just lateral to the pulsations, and 5 mL of solution is injected deep to the fascial plane.

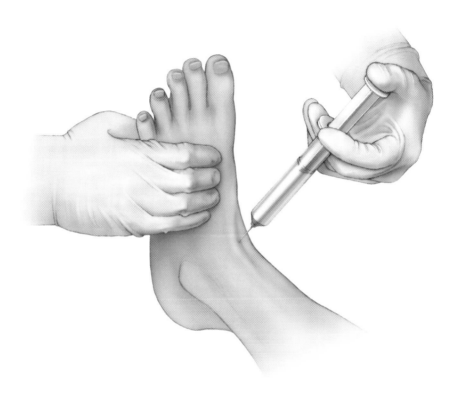

Stabilizing the foot as the deep peroneal nerve is blocked.

Saphenous Nerve Block

Landmarks
The medial malleolus, saphenous vein, and needle insertion site for the deep peroneal nerve block are identified. The saphenous nerve is located between the saphenous vein and the medial malleolus.

Technique
A 25-gauge 3- to 5-cm (1.5- to 2-inch) needle is inserted at the site for the deep peroneal nerve block and directed medially to subcutaneously infiltrate 5 mL of solution around the great saphenous vein.

Superficial Peroneal Block

Landmarks
The insertion site is the same as that for the deep peroneal and saphenous nerve blocks and the lateral malleolus. The superficial peroneal nerve is superficial and medial to the lateral malleolus.

Technique
A 25-gauge 3- to 5-cm (1.5- to 2-inch) needle is inserted at the deep peroneal nerve needle insertion site and directed laterally to subcutaneously infiltrate 5 mL of solution extending from the tibialis anterior tendon to the lateral malleolus.

Sural Nerve Block

Landmarks
The cephalic border of the lateral malleolus and the Achilles tendon are identified.

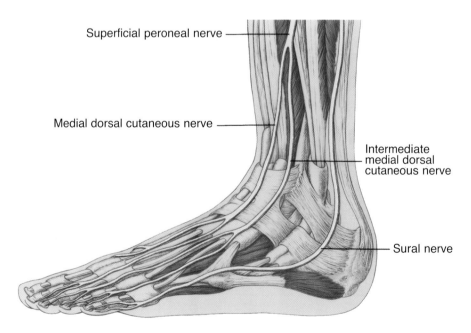

Lateral view of the foot and ankle.

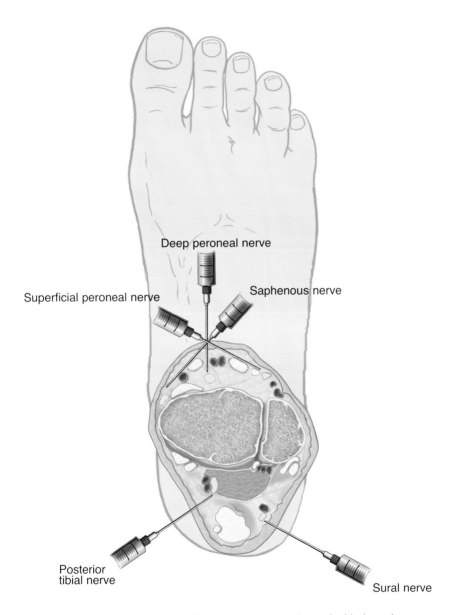

Deep peroneal nerve

Superficial peroneal nerve

Saphenous nerve

Posterior
tibial nerve

Sural nerve

*View of the foot from above. Needle positioning is shown for blocking the
terminal sciatic and saphenous nerves at the level of the malleolus.*

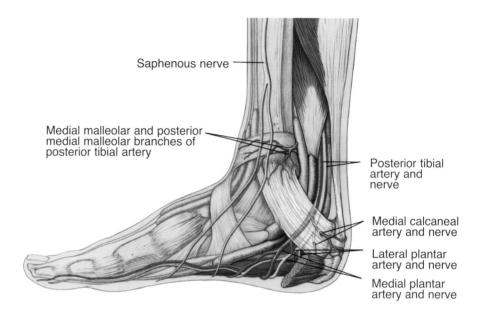

Saphenous nerve

Medial malleolar and posterior medial malleolar branches of posterior tibial artery

Posterior tibial artery and nerve

Medial calcaneal artery and nerve

Lateral plantar artery and nerve

Medial plantar artery and nerve

Medial view of the foot and ankle.

Technique

A 25-gauge 3- to 5-cm (1.5- to 2-inch) needle is inserted between the lateral malleolus and the Achilles tendon and directed anteriorly to inject 5 mL of solution.

Needle Redirection Cues

An alternative is to insert the needle with use of the needle insertion site of the posterior tibial nerve block. The needle passes anterior to the Achilles tendon and is advanced until the needle tip tents the skin, and 5 mL of solution is injected.

Side Effects and Complications

No major complications of ankle block have been reported. Neuropathy and neural ischemia may result from the use of highly concentrated local anesthetic solutions, the use of epinephrine-containing solutions, and the injection of large volumes. Persistent tingling is reported in 2% to 25% of patients postoperatively, but it is presumed that the majority of these cases are related to the surgical procedure or tourniquet ischemia.

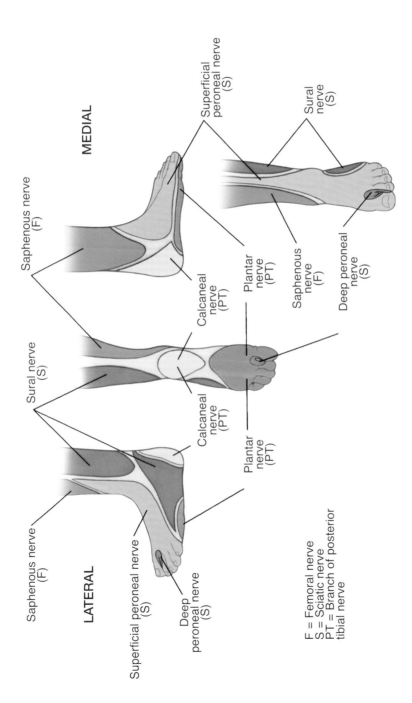

Sensory distribution of the foot and ankle.

Recommended Reading

Colgrove RC. Posterior tibial nerve block. Foot Ankle Int. 2001;22:839-40.

Gerbert J. The location of the terminal branching of the posterior tibial nerve and its effect on administering a posterior tibial nerve block. J Am Podiatry Assoc. 1971;61:8-11.

Needoff M, Radford P, Costigan P. Local anesthesia for postoperative pain relief after foot surgery: a prospective clinical trial. Foot Ankle Int. 1995;16:11-3.

Schurman DJ. Ankle-block anesthesia for foot surgery. Anesthesiology. 1976;44:348-52.

MAYO CLINIC
ANALGESIC PATHWAY

Chapter 20

MAYO CLINIC TOTAL JOINT ANESTHESIA AND ANALGESIC PATHWAY

Patients who undergo total joint arthroplasty experience significant postoperative pain. Failure to provide adequate analgesia impedes aggressive physical therapy and rehabilitation, which is critical to maintaining joint range of motion, and potentially delays hospital dismissal. Traditionally, analgesia after total joint replacement was provided by either intravenous patient-controlled analgesia or epidural analgesia. However, each technique has distinct advantages and disadvantages. For example, opioids do not consistently provide adequate pain relief and often cause sedation, constipation, nausea or vomiting, and pruritus. Epidural infusions containing local anesthetics (with or without an opioid) provide superior analgesia but are associated with hypotension, urinary retention, motor block that limits ambulation, and hematoma due to anticoagulation.

Recently, single-dose and continuous peripheral nerve techniques, which block the lumbar plexus (fascia iliaca, femoral, psoas compartment blocks) with or without sciatic nerve blockade, have been used among this patient population. Several European studies have reported that unilateral peripheral block provided a quality of analgesia and surgical outcomes similar to those of continuous epidural analgesia but with fewer side effects. This finding suggests that continuous peripheral techniques may be the optimal analgesic method after total joint arthroplasty.

Historically, total joint arthroplasty was associated with a hospitalization extending nearly 3 weeks. During the past 2 decades, the typical duration of hospitalization progressively decreased (but plateaued) to 4 to 5 days. However, innovations in surgical approach, such as minimally invasive (incision) surgery, and the introduction of multimodal analgesia have increased the patient's ability to participate in physical therapy in the acute postoperative period and have shortened hospital stays by 1 or 2 days. Superior analgesia with minimal (opioid-related) side effects is crucial to perioperative management. Although alternative protocols have involved epidural infusions with supplemental intravenous opioids postoperatively, the Mayo Clinic total joint analgesic pathway approach uses peripheral nerve blockade and oral analgesics.

This pathway is designed as a practical guide. An understanding of the pharmacology of opioid and non-opioid analgesics, anatomy, traditional and novel techniques of neural localization, and methods of neural blockade is crucial to the safe and efficient implementation of this clinical pathway. The clinician is encouraged to consult the standard references provided throughout for a more comprehensive review of these elements.

Perioperative Management

The perioperative management of patients undergoing total joint replacement is divided into preoperative, intraoperative (anesthetic), and postoperative (analgesic) regimens. The rationale for the patient care components, as well as alternatives, is discussed. This patient care pathway is based on the experience of the authors. All patient care decisions remain the responsibility of the attending physicians and may require modification depending on local institutional practices, procedures, and treatment policies. This pathway may be revised as additional information becomes available.

Indications

All patients undergoing primary or revision joint replacement are candidates for the total joint analgesic pathway. Patients with preexisting neurologic deficits, such as spinal stenosis, an active lumbar radiculopathy, sciatic or peroneal neuropathy, or demyelinating disorder must be considered individually. Untreated infection and altered hemostasis are considered relative contraindications to regional blockade.

Although the total joint analgesic pathway was developed for patients undergoing joint replacement, it also can be applied to patients having other major lower extremity procedures such as hip disarticulation, repair of hip fracture, femoral rod placement, and tumor resection. The role of the technique for nonsurgical or medical indications, such as the treatment and prevention of complex pain syndromes, remains unstudied.

Preoperative Period

All patients are scheduled for a preoperative evaluation. Exclusion criteria for the total joint analgesic pathway include contraindications to regional anesthesia (progressive spinal or peripheral nerve disorder, infection at the needle insertion site, anticoagulation with low-molecular-weight heparin, warfarin, or clopidogrel), and allergy to local anesthetics or other joint pathway medications. Although the American Society of Anesthesiologists physical status I or II may facilitate physical therapy, increased age, significant cardiopulmonary disease, and obesity are not considered contraindications. Indeed, ongoing experience suggests that patients with these factors may benefit the most from the total joint pathway and that their hospital course is uncomplicated and proportionally shortened.

The preoperative history and physical examination should include review of the following:

- Medication-related nausea or vomiting
- Drugs affecting coagulation (discontinue in accordance with the American Society of Regional Anesthesia and Pain Medicine Consensus Statements on Neuraxial Anesthesia and Anticoagulation, www.asra.com)
- Neurologic function, with documentation of any preexisting deficits
- Hemoglobin and creatinine levels

The peripheral nerve techniques should be described to the patient, and the patient should be informed that the presence of the blocks postoperatively will decrease his or her ability to, for example, wiggle toes, and that this is a normal effect of the blocks.

Patient Waiting Area

On arrival to the patient waiting area, the following steps are accomplished:

1. Intravenous access is established
2. Oxycodone (sustained-release, 20 mg orally) is administered

These steps should not occur more than 1 hour preoperatively, or the likelihood of nausea or gastric upset is increased.

Regional Anesthesia "Block Area"

Ideally, peripheral blocks are performed in a designated "block area" to decrease operating room time and to allow adequate time for onset of regional blockade. However, this procedure may not be possible in all institutions. The time required to perform lower extremity blocks dramatically decreases with experience, typically requiring less than 15 minutes (from patient positioning to completion of local anesthetic injection) after 25 blocks have been performed.

1. The patient is positioned with the operative side nondependent
2. Sedatives (midazolam 1-2 mg intravenously and fentanyl 50-100 µg intravenously) are administered
3. The total dose of local anesthetic must be monitored carefully. A maximum of 225 mg of bupivacaine or ropivacaine is recommended. Epinephrine should be added to the initial bolus to allow identification of intravascular injection and to decrease systemic levels of local anesthetics

A complete block of the lumbar plexus (femoral, lateral femoral cutaneous, obturator nerves) is accomplished with the psoas block. In comparison, the fascia iliaca and femoral approaches reliably block the femoral but not the lateral femoral cutaneous and obturator nerves. Complete unilateral lower extremity blockade is achieved with a continuous psoas compartment (preferred), femoral, or fascia iliaca block, in combination with a proximal sciatic block. The sciatic block is performed first, because block onset often is protracted compared with lumbar plexus techniques. Selection of regional analgesic technique is dependent on the surgical site:

• Total (or unicompartmental) knee replacement
    Psoas compartment or femoral catheter
    Sciatic single injection block
• Total hip replacement
• Psoas compartment or fascia iliaca catheter

Intraoperative Course

Combined lumbar plexus and sciatic blockade may be sufficient to provide the sole intraoperative anesthesia, if adequate onset time is allowed. However, the regional block typically is supplemented with an intravenous infusion of propofol.

- The airway may be secured with a laryngeal mask airway or endotracheal tube, particularly during the early stages of pathway implementation while the anesthesia and surgical teams are mastering techniques
- Opioid administration is limited to a maximum of 150 to 250 µg of fentanyl. No long-acting opioids (morphine, hydromorphone) are administered
- Normothermia and volume status are maintained to minimize the need for temperature or volume correction in the postoperative anesthesia recovery room
- Antiemetic prophylaxis is administered only to patients with a history of significant postoperative nausea and vomiting. The avoidance of neuraxial or intravenous opioids and general anesthesia places patients at a low risk for postoperative nausea and vomiting; routine use of antiemetic therapy is not warranted

Postoperative Course

Anesthesia Care Unit

Management of the patient in the postoperative anesthesia care unit includes assessment of adequate regional blockade, administration of supplemental analgesics as needed, and correction of temperature and volume status.

- Immediately on arrival to the unit, the patient's vital signs are measured. A warming device is placed or the hemoglobin level is assessed, as appropriate. A target hemoglobin of 10.0 g/dL is considered adequate in the absence of significant cardiopulmonary disease

- The presence of lumbar plexus (anterior thigh numbness and weakness) and sciatic (foot numbness and weakness) block is verified. Negative aspiration of the lumbar plexus catheter is confirmed, and a bolus is administered and infusion initiated:

    Psoas compartment or femoral catheter

    Bolus 10 mL bupivacaine 0.2%

    Infusion bupivacaine 0.2% at 10 mL/h

    Fascia iliaca

    Bolus 20 mL bupivacaine 0.25%

    Infusion bupivacaine 0.1% at 20 mL/h

- A visual analog score more than 4 warrants supplemental analgesia. A combination of oxycodone and acetaminophen (2 tablets orally) is administered. Rarely, intravenous fentanyl (50-100 µg) is needed

Patient Care Unit

Patient management on arrival to the surgical ward is a continuation of that implemented in the postoperative anesthesia care unit. Essentially all analgesic requirements are met with the combination of peripheral nerve block and scheduled administration of oral acetaminophen and sustained-release oxycodone. Only a few patients require additional oral opioids for breakthrough pain. However, a nonfunctional or dislodged lumbar plexus catheter may necessitate intravenous opioids. A responsive anesthesia pain service is required to treat breakthrough pain immediately and effectively. An attentive nursing staff anticipates evolving analgesic requirements as physical therapy and activity increase.

Postoperatively, patients with an inadequate or failed block and patients with opioid dependence may require opioids intravenously (Table 1). Likewise, lower doses or alternative agents may be warranted in patients who are opioid-intolerant (Table 2).

- Oral intake should be encouraged (and rapidly advanced) to decrease nausea associated with oral analgesics
- Scheduled oral analgesics:

    Oxycodone 10 mg orally at 0800 and 2000 for patients 70 years or older

    Oxycodone 20 mg orally at 0800 and 2000 for patients younger than 70 years (use of oxycodone may be discontinued after 48 hours to avoid sedation and other opioid-related side effects)

Table 1. Intravenous Opioids for Patient-Controlled Analgesia[*]

Agent	Bolus	Lockout interval, min	4-Hour maximal dose	Infusion rate
Fentanyl, 10 µg/mL	10-20 µg	5-10	300 µg	20-100 µg/h
Hydromorphone, 0.2 mg/mL	0.1-0.2 mg	5-10	3 mg	0.1-0.2 mg/h
Meperidine, 10 mg/mL	5-25 mg	5-10	200 mg[†]	5-15 mg/h[†]
Morphine sulfate, 1 mg/mL	0.5-2.5 mg	5-10	30 mg	1-10 mg/h

[*]*Intravenous administration of opioids should be minimized. An intravenous patient-controlled analgesic regimen is typically required only if a peripheral block is inadequate or incomplete or the patient is opioid-dependent.*

[†]*Meperidine limit in healthy patients should be 800 mg in the first 24 hours, then 600 mg every 24 hours thereafter.*

Acetaminophen, 1,000 mg orally at 0800, 1200, and 1600 (maximal acetaminophen dose of 4,000 mg/d from all sources should not be exceeded)
• Supplemental analgesics:
Oxycodone 5 to 10 mg orally every 4 hours as needed: 5 mg if patient complains of pain and rates pain score less than 4; 10 mg if pain score is 4 or more
Ketorolac 15 mg intravenously every 6 hours as needed for four doses. Ketorolac should not be administered to patients with renal insufficiency or patients receiving thromboprophylaxis with low-molecular-weight heparin, warfarin, or aspirin
• Lumbar plexus infusions:
Pain service rounds should be made in the morning to optimize analgesia for the upcoming day. Patients should be educated as to the oral analgesic regimen, including the option of additional medications for breakthrough pain. Reassurance regarding residual sciatic block may be necessary
Psoas compartment or femoral infusion

Table 2.   Oral Analgesics

Drug[*]	Analgesic dose[†]	Dosing interval	Maximal daily dose	Comments
Acetaminophen	500-1,000 mg	q 4-6 h	4,000 mg	As effective as aspirin; 1,000 mg more effective than 650 mg in some patients
Nonsteroidal anti-inflammatory drugs				
Celecoxib (Celebrex)	400 mg initially, then 200 mg	q 12 h		Celecoxib is the only cyclooxygenase-2 inhibitor available in North America; Valdecoxib and rofecoxib recently were removed from the market because of concerns about cardiovascular risk
Aspirin	325-1,000 mg	q 4-6 h	4,000 mg	Most potent antiplatelet effect
Ibuprofen (Advil, Motrin, Nuprin, others)	200-400 mg	q 4-6 h	3,200 mg	200 mg equal to 650 mg aspirin or acetaminophen
Naproxen (Aleve, Naprosyn, others)	500 mg	q 12 h	1,000 mg	250 mg equal to 650 mg aspirin, but with longer duration
Ketorolac (Toradol)	15-30 mg IM/IV	q 4-6 h	60 mg (≥65 years); 120 mg (<65 years)	Comparable to 10 mg morphine; reduce dose in patients <50 kg or with renal impairment; total duration of administration is 5 days
Opioids				
Oxycodone (Oxycontin)	10-20 mg	q 12 h		Limit to total of four doses to avoid accumulation and opioid-related side effects
Controlled-release morphine (MS Contin)	15-30 mg	q 8-12 h		Limit to total of four doses to avoid accumulation and opioid-related side effects

Table 2 (continued)

Drug*	Analgesic dose†	Dosing interval	Maximal daily dose	Comments
Opioids (continued)				
Oxycodone (Roxicodone)	5-10 mg	q 4-6 h		Combination products‡ of oxycodone/acetamino-phen (Percocet, Tylox) and oxycodone-aspirin (Percodan) also are available
Hydromorphone (Dilaudid)	2-4 mg	q 4-6 h		Also available as suppository (3 mg) with 6-8 h effect
Hydrocodone (Lortab, Vicodin, Zydone)	5-10 mg	q 4-6 h		All preparations contain acetaminophen‡
Codeine	30-60 mg	q 4 h		Combination products‡ of codeine-acetamino-phen (Tylenol #2, Tylenol #3, Tylenol #4) and codeine-aspirin (Empirin with codeine) also are available
Propoxyphene (Darvon)	50-100 mg	q 4-6 h	600 mg	Combination products‡ of propoxyphene-acetaminophen (Darvocet, Propoxacet, Tylenol #4) and propoxyphene-aspirin also are available
Tramadol (Ultram)	50-100 mg	q 6 h	400 mg; decrease in cases of renal or hepatic insufficiency	Combination product‡ of tramadol-acetaminophen (Ultracet) also available

IM, intramuscularly; IV, intravenously; q, every.

*Brand names of drugs are in parentheses.

†All doses are oral unless specified otherwise.

‡Dose in combination products is limited by acetaminophen or aspirin ingestion.

Infusion of bupivacaine 0.2% at 10 mL/h is continued until 0600 the day after operation. At 0600 the day after operation, bupivacaine 0.1% at 12 mL/h is given for 24 hours. (Bupivacaine concentration is decreased from 0.2% to 0.1% to ensure that complete weight bearing is possible. After conversion to bupivacaine 0.1%, a detectable block may not be reported)

Fascia iliaca infusion

Continuous infusion bupivacaine 0.1% at 20 mL/h for 48 hours

Dismissal prescriptions consist of oxycodone with acetaminophen; patients are not dismissed with Oxycontin.

Chapter 21

Regional Anesthesia and Analgesia in the Patient Receiving Thromboprophylaxis

As medical standards for the prevention of perioperative venous thromboembolism have been established, new challenges have arisen in the management of patients having orthopedic surgery and neuraxial and peripheral blocks. Patients undergoing major orthopedic surgery, including hip and knee arthroplasty and repair of hip fracture, are at particularly high risk for venous thromboembolism. Routine thromboprophylaxis has been the standard of care for nearly 2 decades. The most recent recommendations of the American College of Chest Physicians regarding prevention of thromboembolism in patients undergoing total joint replacement or repair of hip fracture include three anticoagulant regimens:

- Low-molecular-weight heparin (LMWH) therapy started 12 hours preoperatively, or 12 to 24 hours postoperatively, or 4 to 6 hours postoperatively at half the usual dose and the dose is increased to the usual high-risk dose the following day
- Fondaparinux (2.5 mg 6-8 hours postoperatively)
- Adjusted-dose warfarin started preoperatively or the evening after operation (target international normalized ratio [INR], 2.5; INR range, 2.0-3.0)

Intermittent pneumatic compression is an alternative to anticoagulant prophylaxis in patients undergoing total knee (but not hip) replacement.

The recent introduction of more efficacious anticoagulants and antiplatelet agents has further increased the complexity of patient management. Anesthesiologists must balance the risk of thromboembolic and hemorrhagic complications. Although spinal hematoma remains the most significant hemorrhagic complication of regional anesthesia because of the catastrophic nature of bleeding into a fixed and noncompressible space, the associated risk after plexus and peripheral techniques remains undefined. Clinicians must be aware of the coagulation status of the patient not only at the time of needle or catheter placement but also during catheter maintenance and removal.

In response to these patient safety issues, the American Society of Regional Anesthesia and Pain Medicine developed its Consensus Statements on Neuraxial Anesthesia and Anticoagulation (www.asra.com). The current information focuses on neuraxial blocks and anticoagulants. Conservatively, these neuraxial guidelines may be applied to plexus and peripheral techniques. However, they may be more restrictive than necessary.

Preoperative Anticoagulant and Antiplatelet Agents

With the exception of nonsteroidal anti-inflammatory drugs, the effects of preoperative warfarin, LMWH, standard heparin, or thienopyridine derivatives (clopidogrel, ticlopidine) should be allowed to resolve before regional block.

In patients who are therapeutically anticoagulated preoperatively because of a mechanical heart valve, hypercoagulability, or recent thromboembolic event, aggressive anticoagulation is done postoperatively, when the risk of subsequent thromboembolic complications further increases. The timing of the first anticoagulant dose and the degree of anticoagulation should be discussed with the surgeon preoperatively to determine anesthetic and analgesic management.

Postoperative Management and Removal of Plexus and Peripheral Catheters

Spinal hematoma was considered a rare complication of neuraxial blockade until the introduction of LMWH as a thromboprophylactic agent in the 1990s. The calculated incidence (approximately 1 in 3,000 uses of epidural anesthetics) and the catastrophic nature of spinal bleeding (only 30% of patients had good neurologic recovery) warranted an alternative approach to analgesic management after total hip and knee replacement. Although psoas compartment and femoral catheters are suitable (if not superior) alternatives to neuraxial infusions, no investigations have examined the frequency and severity of hemorrhagic complications after plexus or peripheral blockade in anticoagulated patients. Of reassurance, there are few reports of serious complications after neurovascular sheath cannulation for surgical, radiologic, or cardiac indications. For example, during interventional cardiac procedures, large-bore catheters are placed within brachial or femoral vessels and heparin, LMWH, antiplatelet medications, or thrombolytics subsequently are administered. Despite the significant vessel trauma and coagulation deficiencies, neurologic complications are rare (although a blood transfusion occasionally is required). Thus, although bleeding into a neurovascular sheath may result in significant decreases in hematocrit values, the expandable nature of a peripheral site may decrease the chance of irreversible neural ischemia.

Several cases of vascular injury (with or without resultant nerve dysfunction) have been described in patients with normal and abnormal hemostasis. However, all cases of major bleeding (significant decreases in hemoglobin level or blood pressure) associated with nonneuraxial techniques occurred after psoas compartment or lumbar sympathetic blockade and involved heparin, LMWH, warfarin, and thienopyridine derivatives. These cases suggest that significant blood loss, rather than neural deficits, may be the most serious complication of nonneuraxial regional techniques in the anticoagulated patient. Additional information is needed to make definitive recommendations. The following American Society of Regional Anesthesia and Pain Medicine Consensus Statements on Neuraxial Anesthesia and Anticoagulation may be applied to plexus and peripheral techniques. However, this approach may be more conservative than necessary for superficial and compressible sites, such as the femoral sheath.

- LMWH: Needle placement should occur 10 to 12 hours after a dose. Indwelling neuraxial catheters are allowed with once-daily (but not twice-daily) dosing of LMWH. In general, the optimal technique is to place or remove indwelling catheters in the morning and administer LMWH in the evening to allow normalization of hemostasis before catheter manipulation
- Warfarin: Levels of all vitamin-K–dependent factors should be adequate during catheter placement and removal. Patients chronically receiving warfarin should have normal INR before performance of regional technique. Prothrombin time and INR should be monitored daily. The catheter is removed when the INR is less than 1.5
- Fondaparinux: Neuraxial techniques are not advised in patients who are anticipated to receive fondaparinux perioperatively
- Nonsteroidal anti-inflammatory drugs: No significant risk of regional anesthesia-related bleeding is associated with aspirin-type drugs. However, for patients receiving warfarin or LMWH, the combined anticoagulant and antiplatelet effects may increase the risk of perioperative bleeding.

Thromboembolism is a serious complication of total joint replacement. The development of new antithrombotic drugs, mechanical devices, and postoperative rehabilitation regimens is paramount for improving patient outcome. Peripheral techniques, which allow for early ambulation and earlier hospital dismissal, may prove to be an integral component of patient care. However, currently, they do not replace the need for pharmacologic thromboprophylaxis.

Recommended Reading

Capdevila X, Barthelet Y, Biboulet P, Ryckwaert Y, Rubenovitch J, d'Athis F. Effects of perioperative analgesic technique on the surgical outcome and duration of rehabilitation after major knee surgery. Anesthesiology. 1999;91:8-15.

Geerts WH, Pineo GF, Heit JA, Bergqvist D, Lassen MR, Colwell CW, et al. Prevention of venous thromboembolism: the Seventh ACCP Conference on Antithrombotic and Thrombolytic Therapy. Chest. 2004;126 Suppl:338S-400S.

Horlocker TT. Thromboprophylaxis and neuraxial anesthesia. Orthopedics. 2003;26 Suppl:s243-9.

Horlocker TT, Wedel DJ, Benzon H, Brown DL, Enneking FK, Heit JA, et al. Regional anesthesia in the anticoagulated patient: defining the risks (the second ASRA Concensus Conference on Neuraxial Anesthesia and Anticoagulation). Reg Anesth Pain Med. 2003;28:172-97.

Maier C, Gleim M, Weiss T, Stachetzki U, Nicolas V, Zenz M. Severe bleeding following lumbar sympathetic blockade in two patients under medication with irreversible platelet aggregation inhibitors. Anesthesiology. 2002;97:740-3.

Weller RS, Gerancher JC, Crews JC, Wade KL. Extensive retroperitoneal hematoma without neurologic deficit in two patients who underwent lumbar plexus block and were later anticoagulated. Anesthesiology. 2003;98:581-5.

Chapter 22

MANAGEMENT OF INPATIENT PERIPHERAL NERVE CATHETERS

Effective postoperative pain management with peripheral nerve blocks and multimodal oral agents is dependent on successful nerve blocks and careful catheter placement. Equally important is competent and committed management of indwelling peripheral nerve catheters during hospitalization. Catheter failure due to dislodgement or occlusion is dispiriting to the patient and discouraging to the attending caregivers. Care in securing the catheter hub and diligently placing the catheter dressing at the time of placement decrease the number of unscheduled catheter evaluations at the bedside and may be the difference between success or failure. The catheter site must be inspected daily and the catheter dressing reinforced as needed.

Patients are evaluated daily for the presence and effectiveness of peripheral nerve blockade throughout their hospital stay. Assessment occurs after the block is performed in the block area or operating room, on the patient's arrival in the postoperative anesthesia care unit, and on a daily basis.

Nerve Block Assessment

Neal described a simple and effective system for assessing the effectiveness of lower extremity blocks. PUSH, PULL, PINCH, PUNT is a useful, simple, easy-to-learn method of assessing lower extremity blocks.

Sciatic Nerve

PUSH: The patient is asked to push against the examiner's hand or "to step on the gas" with his or her foot. This push method evaluates the adequacy of sciatic nerve block.

Obturator Nerve
PULL: The examiner abducts the patient's thigh and asks the patient to pull his or her thigh to the midline. This pull method evaluates the obturator nerve block by testing the strength of the adductors of the thigh.

Lateral Femoral Cutaneous Nerve
PINCH: The examiner pinches the skin on the lateral proximal thigh. This pinch method evaluates the lateral femoral nerve block.

Femoral Nerve
PUNT: The examiner supports the patient's knee, lifting it off the bed, and asks the patient to punt an imaginary football. This punt method evaluates femoral nerve block by testing the strength of the quadriceps contraction to extend the leg.

Inadequate Analgesia

The first step in the management of inadequate analgesia is to assess the effectiveness of the nerve blocks and inspect the catheter insertion site. If the catheter appears to be secure (and has not been obviously dislodged), a test bolus dose of local anesthetic is administered to reassess the effectiveness of the block. If appropriate sensory block occurs, correct catheter placement is confirmed.

If after the test bolus the patient reports adequate (improved) analgesia, insufficient volume or dose of local anesthetic likely was the cause of inadequate pain relief and the infusion rate is increased.

If assessment reveals no increase in sensory block, the catheter is no longer in the appropriate location. The catheter is removed and a decision must be made regarding replacement of a similar catheter or selection of an alternative technique. For example, although the fascia iliaca block is not as effective as the psoas approach for blocking the lumbar plexus, a rescue fascia iliaca catheter is a suitable option when it is difficult to reposition the patient (e.g., after hip surgery). Also, it may be prudent, if the femoral nerve is partially blocked, to replace a nonfunctional femoral nerve catheter with a fascia iliaca catheter (theoretically, less risk of nerve injury). As a last resort, another mode of analgesic therapy can be chosen.

Blood Aspiration

Aspiration of frank blood through the peripheral catheter indicates vessel cannulation. However, aspiration of slightly blood-tinged local anesthetic does not necessarily mean venous cannulation. (Likewise, a negative aspiration does not guarantee that the catheter is extravascular.)

The first step in the management of blood aspiration is to inject a small amount of normal saline and reaspirate. If frank blood again is aspirated, the catheter is withdrawn until blood flow stops. The catheter is then reinjected with saline and reaspirated to verify the absence of heme.

For more definitive confirmation of an extravascular location, a 3-mL test dose of saline containing epinephrine 1:200,000 may be injected. An increase in the systolic blood pressure or pulse 20% from baseline indicates that the catheter is intravascular and must be removed. Patients receiving β-adrenergic antagonists may *not* respond with an increase in heart rate. However, the systolic blood pressure will increase.

Catheter Entrapment

Most catheters are removed intact with deliberate, firm, steady traction. Rarely does removal of the catheter prove difficult. Catheter entrapment usually is due to catheter kinking or knotting. Should this occur, the situation is frankly discussed with the patient, including the possiblity of nerve injury and a retained catheter fragment, as well as the potential need for surgical or radiologic intervention.

The technique to help facilitate the removal of an entrapped catheter is dependent on the type of catheter placement. For removal of an entrapped psoas catheter, the patient is placed in the position used for catheter placement and a firm, steady pull technique is used, similar to that for removal of an epidural catheter.

In contrast, this approach may deter the removal of an entrapped femoral or fascia lata catheter; placing the patient in the supine position conceptually "tightens" the fascial planes, making removal of a kinked or knotted catheter much more difficult. Flexion of the ipsilateral hip "loosens" the fascial planes and facilitates removal of an entrapped catheter. Thus, for removal of an entrapped fascia iliaca or femoral catheter, the patient is seated with the ipsilateral hip flexed. The catheter is pulled with firm, steady traction.

Traction should cease if the catheter begins to attenuate, otherwise breakage will occur. Subsequent consultation with an interventional radiologist or surgeon is recommended to determine the optimal method for catheter removal.

No definitive recommendation can be made regarding the removal of a retained fragment. Because neural catheters are inert, they are typically left in situ and the patient is advised to return if pain or infection is noted.

Recommended Reading

Bergman BD, Hebl JR, Kent J, Horlocker TT. Neurologic complications of 405 consecutive continuous axillary catheters. Anesth Analg. 2003;96:247-52.

Gozal D, Gozal Y, Beilin B. Removal of knotted epidural catheters. Reg Anesth. 1996;21:71-3.

Hubner T, Gerber H. Knotting of a catheter in the plexus brachialis: a rare complication [German]. Anaesthesist. 2003 Jul;52:606-7. Epub 2003 Jul 10.

Moore DC, Batra MS. The components of an effective test dose prior to epidural block. Anesthesiology. 1981;55:693-6.

Motamed C, Bouaziz H, Mercier FJ, Benhamou D. Knotting of a femoral catheter. Reg Anesth. 1997;22:486-7.

Neal JM. Assessment of lower extremity nerve block: reprise of the Four P's acronym. Reg Anesth Pain Med. 2002;27:618-20.

Chapter 23

Management of Ambulatory Peripheral Nerve Catheters

Outpatient postoperative analgesia after moderately invasive surgery about the knee, such as repair of the anterior cruciate ligament and unicompartmental knee replacement, is provided by continuous femoral nerve block infusion and supplemental oral analgesic medications.

The femoral catheter is placed preoperatively and a bolus of 30 mL of 0.5% bupivacaine is given. Patients undergoing unicompartmental knee replacement also undergo a single-injection sciatic block. Intraoperative anesthetic management may consist of a low-dose spinal (6-7 mg 0.5% bupivacaine) or a fast-track general anesthetic. On arrival in the postoperative anesthesia care unit, the analgesic pathway is implemented: an infusion of 0.1% bupivacaine at 10 mL/h is initiated, breakthrough pain is treated with ketorolac, oxycodone, or combination of oxycodone-acetaminophen, and the patient is educated regarding management of an indwelling femoral catheter and infusion pump.

Patient Education

The patient is informed that the infusion will continue for approximately 48 hours and that use of the catheter and infusion pump will be discontinued and the catheter and pump will be removed and disposed of at that time. Adverse events are reviewed and physician contact information and a set of instructions (see below) are given to the patient. The patient and family are encouraged to discuss their understanding of how the pain will be managed, and any questions and concerns are addressed directly in a competent and compassionate manner. Patients are informed that postoperative pain management is monitored by telephone at 24 and 48 hours. The patient's home telephone number is verified.

Instructions for Use of At-Home Continuous Infusion System

Your postoperative pain is being managed, in part, with a continuous nerve block infusion system. The pump is attached to a catheter (small tube) in your groin which has been placed under the skin and next to a nerve that supplies the area where your operation was performed. The pump automatically delivers the medicine at a slow flow rate. Listed below is some important information regarding the pain pump.

Drug solution: The solution contained within your pump is bupivacaine 0.1%, and it is being infused at a rate of 10 mL/h. It will take approximately 48 hours for your pump to empty completely. This information is important and should be provided to any health care provider who inquires about its contents.

Catheter information: The local anesthetic initially will make your leg numb. Over time, this degree of numbness will decrease, but usually your leg is not normal until the catheter is removed. Because your leg will not function normally, YOU SHOULD NOT WALK WITHOUT ASSISTANCE, OR DRIVE UNTIL AFTER THE CATHETER HAS BEEN REMOVED.

Complications that could occur include the following:

- The catheter may fall out. If this occurs, make sure to take your pain medicine and turn off the pump.
- Fluid may leak around the catheter. You can change or reinforce the dressing if necessary.
- The catheter may migrate into a blood vessel and cause high levels of local anesthetic. If you experience any of the side effects noted below, close the clamp on the infusion pump system and notify your physician immediately:

Drowsiness	Blurred vision	Poor balance
Dizziness	Slurred speech	Tingling around the mouth or lips

Catheter removal: After the prescribed infusion time has passed (approximately 48 hours), the pain pump should be nearly empty. At that time:
1. Close the clamp on the infusion pump system
2. Remove from your groin all the tape that surrounds the catheter
3. Gently pull the nerve catheter out from its location under the skin. The catheter should slide out easily without pain or resistance. If pain or resistance occurs, notify your physician
4. Confirm that a small black dot is at the tip of the catheter. If this is not present, notify your physician
5. Discard the catheter, the entire pain pump, and all its tubing

Physician contact: If you have any questions or concerns regarding your continuous nerve block infusion system, or if you experience any of the side effects described above, contact your physician for medical assistance.

Postoperative Assessment of Pain Management

At 24 and 48 hours, a nurse from the acute pain service calls the patient to assess pump function and postoperative pain management. The level of sedation, side effects, presence of nausea or emesis, the character and intensity of pain (at rest and movement), and the need for supplemental analgesics are documented in the patient's medical record. The patient also is questioned regarding extremity numbness, catheter site discomfort, and symptoms of local anesthetic toxicity. The assigned physician is informed of the patient's condition.

Chapter 24

Nursing Management of Peripheral Nerve Catheters

Local anesthetic is infused around nerves to control pain. This technique is also known as continuous regional analgesia. Although peripheral nerve catheters are placed by anesthesiologists, nursing contributions are critical to the safe and efficacious management of peripheral nerve infusions.

Principles of medication administration include:

- Medications administered by peripheral nerve catheters are ordered by anesthesiologists or a member of an inpatient pain service and are supplied by the pharmacy
- Medications used for peripheral nerve administration are preservative-free and diluted in normal saline
- Peripheral nerve medications should be clearly labeled with the specific catheter route and infused with a designated regional anesthesia pump

Nursing Assessment

Nursing assessments of the peripheral nerve catheter need to be conducted every 4 hours until use of the nerve catheter is discontinued. Nursing assessment includes:

- Visual inspection of the integrity of the infusion tubing, peripheral nerve catheter, connector between nerve catheter and infusion tubing, and sterile dressing over the catheter insertion site
- Subjective and objective evaluation of the patient's pain experience, including the location, quality, and intensity

- Neurologic evaluation of the upper and lower extremities, including strength, movement, and sensation of the affected extremity
- Visual inspection and palpation of the catheter insertion site, noting the presence of erythema, drainage, tenderness, swelling, or induration at the site
- Observation and questioning of the patient for symptoms of local anesthetic toxicity. Symptoms of local anesthetic toxicity, in increasing order of severity, are circumoral or tongue numbness or tingling sensation, metallic taste in the mouth, tinnitus, restlessness, irritability, excitation, confusion, and seizures

Resources
The inpatient pain service follows patients who have peripheral nerve catheters for 24 hours a day for the duration of the need for the catheter for pain control. In addition, nurses on the inpatient pain service are available by pager from 0700 to 1700 Monday through Friday for answering questions regarding patient care, troubleshooting catheter management issues, removing catheters, and providing education to staff nurses. The inpatient pain service should be called under the following conditions:

- Any significant change in assessment findings
- Break in the integrity of the catheter to the connector or sterile dressing over the insertion site
- Uncontrolled pain
- Increased weakness, changes, or loss of sensation in the extremities
- Signs of infection at insertion site
- Presence of symptoms of local anesthetic toxicity

Chapter 25

FUTURE DIRECTIONS

The art and science of regional anesthesia progressed significantly during the last century, resulting in improved safety and increased success rates. The frequency of serious complications related to neural blockade continues to decrease and is similar, if not superior, to that of general anesthesia. Improved methods of neural localization and imaging such as fluoroscopy, high-resolution ultrasonography, and stimulating catheters have facilitated accurate needle and catheter placement. Most importantly, prospective randomized clinical investigations have found improved outcomes for patients undergoing major surgical procedures when regional anesthesia and analgesia are utilized.

However, an understanding of anatomical relationships, neural innervation, and physiology remains paramount in the application of regional anesthetic and analgesic techniques. Many clinicians do not have ready access to an anatomy laboratory. Classic anatomical atlases were constructed by anatomists, not regional anesthesiologists, resulting in illustrations that depict neural anatomy with the "wrong" limb orientation or cross-sectional view. Finally, the majority of resident training programs do not provide formal training in peripheral blockade. Experienced clinicians and trainees must have access to anatomical sections and simulators, allowing the proceduralist to explore the anatomical relationships between nerves and related structures before patient contact.

Continuous peripheral nerve blocks are an integral part of a multimodal approach to postoperative analgesia after major orthopedic surgery. Additional research is needed to complete our understanding of the ideal delivery devices and infusates. Further efforts to prolong analgesia may include improved drug design, such as controlled-release local anesthetics or innovative additives. Future research should be directed toward improving the ease of performance to increase success (and acceptance). These techniques clearly have a wider application for postoperative pain relief. We envision a future in which peripheral nerve blocks for the lower extremity are widely taught and applied by all anesthesiologists, not just enthusiasts of regional anesthesia.

INDEX

Index